Gluten Free Diet Cookbook: Healthier Eating Choices for People with Celiac Disease

By Maria Holmes

Table of Contents

Preface

Dear Reader!

I would like to take this opportunity to thank you for taking the time to read my book and hope that you find these gluten-free recipes delightful and easy to make!

Before we start exploring how you can prepare amazing gluten-free meals, I would like to introduce myself. My name is Maria Holmes and I am indeed the author of this cookbook that you are now reading. If you are interested in learning more about me, my mission and my passion, please join my Facebook community at Homes Cooked Meals for interesting activities and enthusiastic discussions. Or you might want to visit my blog at www.holmescookedmeals.com.

But let's get back to the topic at hand – *Gluten Free Diet Cookbook: Healthier Eating Choices for People with Celiac Disease.*

I wrote this cookbook out of necessity. My husband was recently diagnosed with Celiac Disease and I found myself learning as much as I could about gluten free cooking. Since going gluten free is the primary means to manage the disease symptoms, I learned to adapt many of my recipes to fit his new diet. My aim is to still keep my recipes as simple as possible without sacrificing taste and good nutrition.

While living a gluten free lifestyle, on a gluten free diet, can have its challenges, I know you can still enjoy satisfying and healthy meals. I hope that you find the 60 gourmet recipes that I am sharing delicious as well as adhering to your dietary restrictions.

So get ready to discover some delightful recipes for people with Celiac Disease, gluten intolerance, food allergies and sensitivities.

Enjoy and be well!

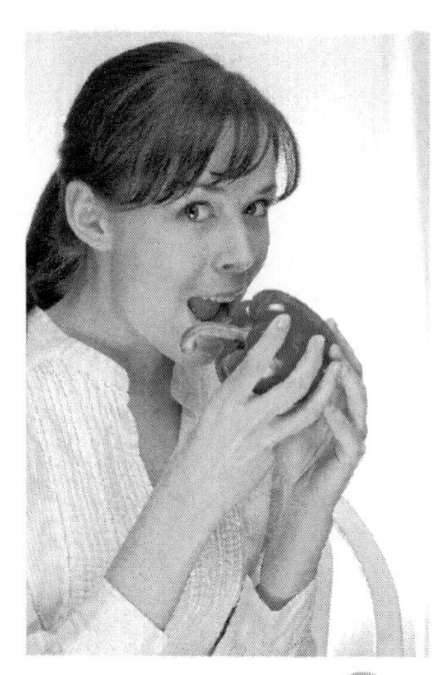

Maria Holmes

Acknowledgement

I would like to express my gratitude to my parents who have always supported and encouraged me in everything I have done in my life. Without their love and support this book might never have been written.

I am also grateful to my dear friends who I often use as test subjects when developing my recipes. Without their help and sacrifice, many of these recipes may have turned out bland and tasteless. Many of these friends have become members and supporters of my Facebook Page and www.holmescookedmeals.com website.

And a special thank you goes out to my loving husband and my two amazing children (Ellie an Isaac) who endlessly encourage me to share my love for food and my many recipes with the world.

And most importantly, thank you, dear reader, for purchasing *Gluten Free Diet Cookbook: Healthier Eating Choices for People with Celiac Disease.*

Managing Gluten Anxiety

Gluten intolerance can be a lifelong challenge and a major stressor whether you've just been diagnosed r have been gluten free for decades. In particular, anxiety is a normal and expected response to the diagnosis of Celiac Disease, which is a chronic condition. Although it is perfectly normal, there are ways to cope with these negative feelings an maintain a happy life that balances health and enjoyment. Luckily, going gluten free is the only treatment you need and, with the right coping skills, you can thrive in the gluten free lifestyle.

Anxiety can take many forms, but usually starts in our head. Anxiety is basically a sense of worry about what might happen in the future ("what is the chef added flour to the sauce? Might I have a reaction later on in the middle of the theater?"). Gluten-related anxiety can cause apprehension about eating in public, trying new foods, traveling and participating in many other activities that should be pleasant. Still, that anxiety protects us against experiencing reactions to gluten that are miserable and lead to further health complications.

Anxiety by nature is a normal, basic human emotion. In fact it can be adaptive … think about how useful anxiety can be if you're out in the jungle and see a lion eying you. Having that initial "fight or flight" response can be very useful for escaping with all your limbs intact. In the modern age, we more often experience anxiety participating in social events, performing in front of others or entering a new and unfamiliar situation. For those with Celiac Disease, some anxiety ensures that you understand that there is a real threat and that you take action to protect your health.

However, too much or too little anxiety can be bad for someone with Celiac Disease. You can easily become trapped in a vicious cycle of fear, paranoia and avoidance that only gets stronger as time goes by. Still, too little anxiety can be problematic too. We've all known someone who says they have Celiac Disease but make decisions that aren't good for them. Maybe they don't want to cause any trouble by asking about the food they are ordering, or sometimes they cheat because they're "not that sensitive". This can have very negative health consequences as well.

So what would "good" anxiety look like? Think of coping with your gluten anxiety to be similar to the story of Goldilocks and the Three Bears. We don't want our fear to be too strong (which can be debilitating) or too weak (which could put out health at risk). Instead, we want to find that "just right" level of vigilance that allows us to live our lives while maximizing out health. It's a delicate balance that takes time to master. Ask yourself the questions below and see which answer you relate to most.

Question	Too Little Anxiety	"Just Right" Anxiety	Too Much Anxiety
How often do I worry about being exposed?	"I often forget to check labels or ask questions about my food."	"Every time an unfamiliar food comes my way I worry about the possibility of getting sick."	"I am always worrying about getting gluten in my system, even when I am eating foods I know are definitely gluten-free."
How reasonable are my expectations about being exposed?	"I sometimes convince myself that I can cheat if it's just a little, or if I've been good all week."	"I know that mistakes can happen, but if I do my best, I can protect myself and still have my life."	"I am skeptical of trusting anyone with my food and feel like I always end up exposed if I try new things."
How severe is my anxiety about being exposed?	"It's no big deal if I get exposed to gluten."	"I definitely worry about getting exposed to gluten, but I Know how to deal with it if it happens."	"I panic at the thought of reacting to gluten and completely fall apart if I have an actual exposure."
How does it affect my behavior?	"I often avoid asking questions or checking labels because I don't want to make it a big deal."	"I ask necessary questions about my food and check labels so I'm less likely to be exposed to gluten."	"I avoid eating out or even going to parties because I might get exposed. It's easier to stay at home."

The key to a "just right" level of gluten anxiety comes down to feeling in control of your situation and knowing how to manage your health.

In a recent study conducted in the United Kingdom at the University of Birmingham, people with Celiac Disease who reported better health related quality of life tended to have lower emotional response to their illness and a higher sense of control. Other studies have shown that Celiac patients are most likely to struggle with anxiety and health problems if they feel isolated or uninformed.

If you think you may have too much or too little anxiety about gluten exposure, consider making changes to improve your life. Ask yourself how your quality of life has been affected by too much or too little gluten anxiety and try making changes to your behavior (practicing more vigilance or facing your fears) in small attainable steps. Join your local support group and educate yourself through websites, books, and smart device apps. Try to have open communication with your family and friends about your struggles.

If you are still struggling with channeling your inner Goldilocks, consider trying psychotherapy. A well-trained professional can e very helpful in learning adaptive coping skills for achieving your goals. Look for a therapist who has experience in chronic illness. With a little knowledge and a lot of practice, you can learn to live your life happier and healthier than ever.

"Super" Gluten Free

Super food is a term that everyone has been seeing a lot of lately. It's on heath food blogs, store shelves and product packaging, and is used to describe a food that is believed to have exceptional nutritional value and health benefits. I am all for trying new foods that offer any type of boost in my health, and I'm sure you are too!

But if you are new to a gluten free lifestyle, you may be overwhelmed at the thought of incorporating a food you may never have heard of before into your diet. But learning about the most popular "super foods" on the market is not that difficult, and before you know it, you'll be "super" gluten free.

Super Foods

Chia:

Remember that Chia Pet you got for Christmas a few years ago? You know, that clay figurine filled with chia seeds that sprouted green fur seemingly overnight? Well did you know that those magical little seeds are packed full of omega-3 fatty acids, fiber, protein and antioxidants and are naturally gluten free? Chia seeds are also gaining popularity among athletes because of their hydrating properties. They are often blended into smoothies, sprinkled on salads and yogurts or made into a pudding for a quick breakfast.

Goji Berries:

Goji berries, which are also naturally gluten free, are popping up everywhere, even covered in dark chocolate! They are well deserving of all the attention they are getting since this small red berry packs a big nutritional punch. They are full of antioxidants, which help your body fight free radicals, contain 18 different amino acids, boast more vitamin C by weight than oranges and supply over 20 other trace minerals and vitamins. They taste similar to a cranberry and can be added to cereals or snacked on like raisins. You can often find goji berries in the form of a powder as well, which can be used to add flavor and nutrition to smoothies and desserts.

Cacao:

Cacao is harvested from beans inside the fruit of the cacao tree and is the basis for chocolate. In its natural state, though slightly more bitter than what you may be used to, it offers a chocolate flavor and texture, is high in magnesium and antioxidants and can provide a natural burst of alertness and energy. Often, people trying to wean themselves off of coffee will add this to their smoothies or cereals for a natural pick-me-up.

Spirulina:

Spirulina is blue green algae and is exceptionally high in amino acids, chlorophyll, enzymes and antioxidants. It is however one super food that can take some getting used to because it turns everything it touches the color of swamp water! Don't let this deter you though, because it has a very mild flavor that is easily masked by blended fruit. Spirulina is sold in powder form and just one heaping tablespoon (or more if you like) a day is all you need to reap the benefits of this amazing little algae.

Acai:

Acai is that really hard to pronounce berry that everyone seems to be talking about. In terms of antioxidants, it's the queen of all berries, packing in more than cranberries, raspberries, blackberries, strawberries or blueberries! I see Acai offered most often in powder and juice form. I prefer the powder because it's easily added to dressings, desserts and juices.

Aloe:

Usually we think of aloe as a skin gel that offers sweet relief after we have accidentally fallen asleep on the beach. However, aloe has just as many healing properties when ingested because it contains essential fatty acids enzymes, amino acids, vitamins and minerals. Aloe is said to have natural anti-inflammatory and detoxifying properties and can aid in digestion. Aloe is taken in small amounts and can be blended into smoothies or mixed with juices.

Navitas:

Navitas is a great brand to go with if you'd like to try adding these super foods to your diet. Depending on where you shop, you might encounter other brands as well. Just be sure to check the label to be certain the product only contains the super food you're looking for and no other gluten-containing ingredients.

Making Milk Super

Some people really don't like the idea of drinking cow's milk. Also, it's not uncommon for gluten intolerance to co-exist with other food sensitivities. One of the more common intolerance is to lactose (dairy products). Luckily, your gluten-free cookies and cereals won't have to be eaten dry because there are plenty of non-dairy milk alternatives. Almond, hemp, flax, coconut, soy and rice milks are among the more popular choices. Blue Diamond's Almond Breeze milks are gluten-free, including their delicious chocolate milk flavor. So Delicious is another brand that offers gluten-free coconut and almond milk.

Seaweed Superfood

A great deal of information has been published lately about the benefits of including seaweed in your diet. It may sound a bit strange to us land dwellers, but seaweed truly is packed with vital nutrients like iodine, calcium, magnesium, iron and trace elements. Wakame, nori, dulse, and kombu are a few of the more popular types of seaweed used in salads, sushi rolls, soups and even as a salt substitute. A good brand to try is Eden Foods, which can be found in many mainstream grocery stores.

Natural Sweeteners

We've all read how terrible refined white sugar is and we still eat a lot of it without even realizing! But let's face it, most of us have a sweet tooth and will never quit the sweet stuff cold turkey. However, there are healthier alternatives on the market that will still satisfy you. One of the more popular sweeteners is agave, which is naturally gluten free. Stevia is another smart alternative because, even though it's very sweet, it's actually an herb and has zero glycemic index and zero calories. You can use it in your coffee, in recipes and for anything else that needs a touch of sweet. Coconut sugar is also gaining in popularity because it is low in glycemic and contains potassium, magnesium, zinc and iron. It can also be used as 1:1 cane sugar replacement. Also check out a new addition to the market, monk fruit sweetener. It's all natural and contains no calories.

Things to Watch Out For

Many of these foods are so nutritionally rich they are being incorporated into many products like cereals, granolas, sweets and energy bars. Don't assume that seeing one of these gluten free super foods touted on product packaging means the items is totally gluten free. Always double-check the label so that when you do choose a super food, you're doing your body well!

Tips for Successfully Changing Your Diet and Lifestyle

Nutrition

Nutrition challenges can be great ways to curb cravings, investigate potential allergies and help jumpstart a healthy diet. Most nutrition challenges involve either adding in certain foods or avoiding foods for a specific period of time, usually 30 days. These challenges are meant to be short-term "resets" or tools to aid in lifelong health and as such, they can often be strict.

Before you begin, make sure you have a great support system. A support system is critical for success, especially on those days when the cravings don't seem to end and you find yourself mentally exhausted. Tell your support system what your goals are and ask them to help keep you on track when you need it and celebrate your success with you.

Whether you're trying to heal your gut, figure out potential food allergies or just trying to lose a few pounds, embarking on a nutrition challenge can be daunting. There are several factors to consider including time, foods to include and avoid, and having enough mental energy to stay happy and healthy. There are lunches to pack, dinners out to navigate, and quick snacks needed to help fuel you through the day. Add a busy lifestyle to the mix and it can seem downright impossible. But it doesn't have to be that way! With a little prep and planning, you can save time, energy and be prepared to curb even the toughest cravings.

Make a Plan

When changing what you eat, having a plan is absolutely necessary. Write down what foods you want to include in your diet and what foods you want to avoid and keep it in a visible place. Write down a few items that you anticipate craving (chocolate, wine, cheese, etc…) and make a plan for what you will do when cravings strike. Craving chocolate, but trying to reign in your sweet tooth? Reach for a piece of low sugar fruit like berries, or brew a cup of delicious herbal tea instead. Having a plan in place will help you succeed in beating your cravings and reaching your goals.

Create a Meal Template

Another way to make your nutrition challenge easier is to create a meal template. A meal template is a rough template of approximately what and how much you will eat each day. Take into account how much food you need to fuel you through your day, how many times a day you prefer to eat out, and any specific dietary requirements you may have. For example, my meal template below reflects my need for high levels of healthy fats and proteins for recovery and athletic performance. It also reflects my preference for eating four meals a day and having a large breakfast and slightly smaller meals throughout the day.

Sample Meal Plans	
Meal #1	2 to 3 eggs + 1/2 cup protein + to 2 cups veggies + 1/2 cup berries or apple, + 1/2 cup sweet potato + almond butter or coconut oil
Meal #2	4 ounces protein + 2 to 3 cups veggies + 1/2 avocado
Meal #3	4 ounces protein + 1 to 2 cups veggies + 1/2 cup coconut flakes
Meal #4	6 ounces protein + 2 to 3 cups veggies + 1/2 cup squash or sweet potato + oils/butter
Optional snacks	Coconut milk green smoothie
Post-Workout Snack	Protein shake with almond milk

Plan Your Meals

Now that you know approximately how much and what kind of food you will be eating, you can begin to plan your meals. You can plan each individual meal or perhaps you prefer to just plan out dinners and figure out the rest later.

If you prefer to eat the same or similar things each day, you can shop accordingly. If you prefer to have a little spontaneity in your meals, you can shop for a variety of items, prepare them, and have them on hand. Either way, having a plan can help save you valuable time and money when it comes time to grocery shop and prep your food.

Prepare Your Food

Having a fridge full of prepared food can make even the strictest nutritional challenge doable for the extremely busy individual. Pick a day on the weekend to spend some time in the kitchen chopping, cooking and preparing your food for the week. This can save you valuable time during the week and if you're prepare, you're never left with the hungry-but-nothing-to-eat predicament. Here are few easy make-ahead items:

- Roast a whole chicken
- Wash and chop vegetables for salads and snacks
- Hardboil a dozen eggs
- Make "snack packs" of portable snacks like nuts
- Cook large portions of multi-use items such as rice and beans
- Roast batches of vegetables like squash, Brussels sprouts and broccoli
- Make a hearty soup or stew to have for the week

Put Your Plan Into Action and Track Your Progress

You've prepped and planned; now it's time to put it into action. At first, changing habits can be difficult – there are a lot of things to remember and it may seem like a lot of effort but over time, it will get easier and become more "automatic". Consider tracking your day-to-day progress through a food journal. Tracking your day-to-day meals, moods and feelings can help identify areas of difficulty, ease and where you may need to revise your plan.

When your challenge is over, you can look back and identify potential emotional triggers for cravings, reasons for energy slumps or foods that may have affected you negatively. You can continue to journal when you re-introduce foods back into your diet to see how your body and mind react – this is extremely helpful for figuring out food allergies and intolerances as well!

Even though planning and preparing food may seem like tedious tasks, it can save you valuable time, money and energy when you're busy. So no matter what your goals are when you set out on your nutritional challenge, you can be successful with a little planning, preparation and support.

Drinks

THE RECIPES

Rose & Honey

Makes 1 drink

Ingredients

1 teaspoon honey
6 ounces dry rose wine, chilled
1/8 teaspoon rosewater
2 dashes Angostura bitters*

* Angostura bitters, often simply referred to as *angostura,* is a concentrated bitter made of water, 44.7% alcohol, herbs and spices. It is typically used for flavoring beverages, or (less often) food. Angosutra bitters can be found almost anywhere you can buy liquor.

Directions

Combine all the ingredients, except the bitters, in a large wine glass and gently whisk until the honey is dissolved.

Top with the bitters and serve.

Nutrition per Serving

Calories: 165; Fat: 0.0g; Cholesterol: 0mg; Sodium: 25.mg; Carbohydrates: 11.0g; Fiber: 0.0g; Sugar: 7.6g; Protein: 0.1g

French 75

Makes 1 drink

Ingredients

1 teaspoon sugar
1 tablespoon fresh lemon juice
3 ounces gin
2 ounces champagne
Lemon peel, for garnish

Directions

Combine the sugar, lemon juice, gin and champagne in a chilled shaker and shake to mix.

Pour into a glass and garnish with lemon peel.

Nutrition per Serving

Calories: 287; Fat: 0.1g; Cholesterol: 0mg; Sodium: 5mg; Carbohydrates: 5.1g; Fiber: 0.0g; Sugar: 4.5g; Protein: 0.1g

Whiskey Wine Punch

Makes 1 drink

Ingredients

1 bottle of dry red wine
1/4 cup whiskey
1/4 cup orange juice
Tangerine slices, for garnish

Directions

Combine the red wine, whiskey, and orange juice in a pitcher and chill until cold.

Pour the punch into a cocktail glass and then garnish with a small tangerine slice.

Nutrition per Serving

Calories: 220; Fat: 0.1g; Cholesterol: 0mg; Sodium: 10mg; Carbohydrates: 7.0g; Fiber: 0.0g; Sugar: 3.0g; Protein: 0.4g

Grapefruit Sparkler

Makes 1 drink

Ingredients

Superfine sugar, for rim
2 tablespoons fresh grapefruit juice
1/2 ounce Lillet-Blanc liquor
Champagne or other sparkling dry white wine

Directions

Wet the edge of a champagne glass with water.

Pour the sugar onto a plate and gently place the edge of the glass onto the sugar, turning a few times to coat.

Pour the fresh grapefruit juice and Lillet-Blanc then top with champagne.

Nutrition per Serving

Calories: 120; Fat: 0.0g; Cholesterol: 0mg; Sodium: 0mg; Carbohydrates: 5.0g; Sugar: 1.0g; Fiber: 0.0g; Protein: 0.0g

Lemon Mint Wine Cooler

Makes 1 drink

Ingredients

2 teaspoon sugar
4 mint leaves, torn
Juice of 1 lemon
5 ounces white wine, chilled
Additional mint, for garnish

Directions

Place the sugar and torn mint leaves in the bottom of a cocktail glass and gently muddle with a spoon or muddler until the mint is very fragrant.

Add the lemon juice and stir to dissolve the sugar.

Top with white wine and garnish with mint sprig.

Nutrition per Serving

Calories: 240; Fat: 1.5g; Cholesterol: 0mg; Sodium: 35mg; Carbohydrates: 36.0g; Fiber: 9.0g; Sugar: 9.0g; Protein: 5.0g

Garden Fresh Bloody Mary

Makes 1 smoothie

Ingredients

1 cup diced beets
1 cup diced celery
1 cup diced tomato
Dash of salt
Dash of pepper
1 ounce vodka (optional)
Dash of cayenne pepper or red pepper flakes (optional)

Directions

Process the diced beets, celery and tomato through a juicer then add the spiced and optional 1 ounce of vodka.

Stir and garnish with fresh stalk of celery or celery leaves.

For added spice, add cayenne pepper or red pepper flakes.

Nutrition per Serving

Calories: 187; Fat: 0.8g; Cholesterol: 0mg; Sodium: 390mg; Carbohydrates: 26.5g; Fiber: 7.2g; Sugar: 19.6g; Protein: 5.1g

Wild Berry Mint Smoothie

Makes 2 smoothies

Ingredients

1 cup unsweetened almond milk (or alternative non-dairy milk)
6 ounces fresh blackberries
6 ounces fresh blueberries
4 fresh mint leaves
1 tablespoon agave nectar
1 ounce vodka (optional)

Directions

Add the almond milk, blackberries, blueberries, mint leaves and agave nectar into a blender or food processor then blend until smooth.

Garnish with fresh mint leaves.

Nutrition per Serving

Calories: 240; Fat: 4.0g; Cholesterol: 0mg; Sodium: 180mg; Carbohydrates: 34.0g; Fiber: 10.0g; Sugar: 24.0g; Protein: 3.0g

Creamy Sage & Lemon Smoothie

Makes 2 smoothies

Ingredients

1 cup unsweetened flax milk (or alternative non-dairy milk)
1/2 cup cold water
3/4 cup avocado, diced
3 tablespoons fresh squeezed lemon juice
4 fresh sage leaves
1/4 cup chopped kale
1 tablespoon agave nectar
1 ounce gin (optional)

Directions

Add the flax milk, water, avocado, lemon juice, sage, kale, and agave nectar into a blender or food processor and blend until smooth and creamy.

Serve garnished with fresh sage leaves.

Nutrition per Serving

Calories: 360; Fat: 19.0g; Cholesterol: 0mg; Sodium: 190mg; Carbohydrates: 32.0g; Fiber: 9.0g; Sugar: 19.0g; Protein: 4.0g

Pineapple Rum Lemonade

Makes 1 cocktail

Ingredients

For the Pineapple-Infused Rum

1/2 cup of pineapple, peeled and diced
1 cup of rum

For the Pineapple Rum Lemonade

Juice of 1 lemon
Club soda
Lemon slice (for garnish)

Directions

For the pineapple-infused rum, combine the pineapples and rum in a large airtight container such as a large mason jar and place in a dark cool place. Shake the mason jar a few times a day. Taste periodically and let infuse until the desired flavor is reached or the pineapple has lost most of its color (normally 3 to 5 days).

For each cocktail, combine 1-1/2 ounces of the pineapple-infused rum and the juice from 1 lemon in a cocktail shaker filled with ice and shake vigorously.

Strain into a martini glass and top with club soda.

Garnish with a lemon slice before serving.

Nutrition per Serving

Calories: 120; Fat: 0.0g; Cholesterol: 0mg; Sodium: 0mg; Carbohydrates: 7.0g; Fiber: 0.0g; Sugar: 6.0g; Protein: 0.0g

Watermelon Gin & Tonic

Makes 1 cocktail

Ingredients

For the Watermelon-Infused Gin

1/2 cup of watermelon, peeled, diced and seeds removed
1 cup of gin

For the Gin & Tonic

1 tablespoon simple syrup
Juice of 1/2 lime
Tonic water
Watermelon chunks (for garnish)
Lime slices (for garnish)

Directions

For the watermelon-infused gin, combine the watermelon and gin in a large airtight container such as a large mason jar and place in a dark cool place. Shake the mason jar a few times a day. Taste periodically and let infuse until the desired flavor is reached or the watermelon has lost most of its color (normally 7 to 10 days).

For each cocktail, combine 1-1/2 ounces of the watermelon-infused gin, 1 tablespoon of simple syrup, and the juice of 1/2 a lime in a glass filled with ice then stir well.

Fill the glass with tonic water and garnish with fresh watermelon chunks and a slice of lime.

Nutrition per Serving

Calories: 170; Fat: 0.0g; Cholesterol: 0mg; Sodium: 10mg; Carbohydrates: 19.0g; Fiber: 0.0g; Sugar: 18.0g; Protein: 0.0g

Soups and Salads

THE RECIPES

Vegetable Soup

Makes 8 to 10 servings

Ingredients

2 tablespoons olive oil
1 onion, diced
2 large carrots, cut into rounds
3 celery stalks, sliced
3 cloves garlic, minced
1/2 teaspoon dried thyme
1/2 teaspoon dried parsley
1 bunch kale, de-stemmed and cut in strips
2 cups green peas
2 quarts vegetable stock
2 tablespoons tomato paste
Salt, to taste
Pepper, to taste

Directions

Heat the olive oil in a large, deep pot over medium-high heat then once hot, add the onions, carrots, and celery and sauté until translucent and soft, about 12 to 15 minutes.

Add the garlic, thyme and parsley then sauté until fragrant, about 2 to 3 minutes.

Add the kale and peas and stir to combine.

Add the vegetable stock and tomato paste and bring to a boil.

Reduce the heat and simmer the soup for 30 minutes.

Season the soup to taste with salt and pepper.

Nutrition per Serving

Calories: 100; Fat: 3.5g; Cholesterol: 0mg; Sodium: 460mg; Carbohydrates: 15.0g; Fiber: 4.0g; Sugar: 5.0g; Protein: 4.0g

Creamy Asparagus Soup

Makes 4 servings

Ingredients

2 teaspoons olive oil
2 teaspoons unsalted butter
2 pounds asparagus, trimmed and chopped into large pieces
1/2 cup yellow onion, minced
1/4 teaspoon salt
3 cups low-sodium chicken or vegetable stock
2 tablespoons dry white wine
1/2 to 3/4 cup heavy whipping cream
2 tablespoons freshly squeezed lemon juice
Salt, to taste
Pepper, to taste

Directions

Place the olive oil and butter in a medium-sized pot and heat over medium heat to melt the butter.

Add the asparagus and onion to the pot then sprinkle with the 1/4 teaspoon of salt and sauté for 7 to 10 minutes, or until the vegetables have softened. Remove 12 asparagus tips from the pot and set aside.

Pour the stock and white wine then bring to a simmer and let cook, uncovered, for 10 minutes. Remove from the heat and let cool for about 10 minutes.

Using an immersion blender, purée the soup until smooth and creamy, or if you don't have an immersion blender, place the ingredients in a blender and blend the soup in batches.

Return the soup to the pot and place over medium-low heat then let cook just long enough to warm the soup through.

Stir in the heavy whipping cream and once combined, add in the lemon juice and season to taste with salt and pepper.

To serve, ladle the soup into 4 bowls and top each serving with 3 of the reserved asparagus spears.

Nutrition per Serving

Calories: 163; Fat: 10.1g; Cholesterol: 26mg; Sodium: 595mg; Carbohydrates: 11.7g; Fiber: 5.0g; Sugar: 5.8g; Protein: 8.5g

Ginger Carrot & Fennel Soup

Makes 6 to 8 servings

Ingredients

2 tablespoons olive oil
2 leeks, rinsed well and thinly sliced (white and light green parts only)
1/2 bulb fresh fennel, thinly sliced
3 cups sliced carrot rounds
1/4 teaspoon curry powder
1/4 teaspoon cinnamon
2 cloves garlic, minced
1/4 cup dry white wine
1/2 teaspoon ground ginger
1 quart vegetable stock
Salt, to taste
Pepper, to taste

Directions

Heat the olive oil in a large pot over medium heat, then add the leeks, fennel and carrots and sauté until very soft, about 10 to 15 minutes.

Add the curry powder and cinnamon.

Add the garlic and sauté another 2 to 3 minutes until fragrant.

Add the white wine and gently scrape the bottom of the pot to remove any browned bits.

Add the ground ginger and gently stir to combine.

Add the vegetable stock and bring to a boil, then reduce to a simmer and cook for 15 to 20 minutes.

Shut off the heat and blend with an immersion blender or in batches in a high-powered blender.

Season the soup with salt and pepper to taste.

Nutrition per Serving

Calories: 80; Fat: 3.5g; Cholesterol: 0mg; Sodium: 510mg; Carbohydrates: 11.0g; Fiber: 2.0g; Sugar: 4.0g; Protein: 1.0g

Spicy Tomato Soup

Serves 6 to 8

Ingredients

1-1/2 cups diced carrots
1-1/2 cups minced onions
4 stalks celery, chopped
4 cloves garlic, crushed
1/4 teaspoon salt
1-1/2 tablespoons olive oil
1-1/2 cups chopped roasted red peppers
1/4 teaspoon black pepper
1 tablespoon dried parsley
1 tablespoon dried dill weed
1/4 teaspoon Tobasco sauce or hot sauce, to taste
2 teaspoons gluten free Worcestershire sauce
1 can (16-ounces) tomato paste
2 cans (32-ounces) chopped tomatoes, preferably fire-roasted with liquid
4 cups gluten free vegetable broth
Pinch cayenne pepper (optional)
2 tablespoons honey

Directions

In a soup kettle, sauté the carrots, onions, celery, garlic and salt in the olive oil.

Add the roasted red peppers and continue to cook.

When the onions are well done, add the black peppers, parsley, dill weed, hot sauce, Worcestershire sauce and tomato pastes and stir to combine.

Add the canned tomatoes, vegetable broth and cayenne pepper, if desired.

Add the honey and stir all the ingredients together.

Cover the soup and let simmer for 40 minutes over a low heat.

Turn off the heat and blend all the ingredients together with an immersion blender.
Adjust the seasoning to taste and serve hot.

Nutrition per Serving

Calories: 141; Fat: 3.0g; Cholesterol: 0mg; Sodium: 246mg; Carbohydrates: 28.0g; Fiber: 6.0g; Sugar: 7.1g; Protein: 4.0g

Corn Chowder

Serves 6 to 8

Ingredients

2 cups diced carrots
2 cups diced onions
2 cups diced celery
1-1/2 tablespoons olive oil
2 teaspoons minced garlic
1/4 cup white rice flour
4 to 6 cups gluten free vegetable broth
1 teaspoon thyme
2 bay leaves
1/2 teaspoon salt
1/2 teaspoon pepper
2 tablespoons chopped parsley
6 to 8 cups corn kernels
2 cups sweet potatoes, peeled and chopped (about 2 large sweet potatoes)
3 tablespoons honey
3/4 cup sunflower seed butter or cashew butter

Directions

Sauté the carrots, onions and celery in the olive oil over a low heat for 10 to 15 minutes.

Add the garlic and cook for another 5 minutes.

Stir in the rice flour and slowly add the vegetable broth.

Add the thyme, bay leaves, salt, pepper, parsley, and corn kernels.

Add the chopped sweet potatoes and honey.

Bring the soup to a boil and then turn the heat down to a simmer.

Add the sunflower seed butter and mix thoroughly.

Let the soup simmer, covered, for an additional 45 minutes.

Remove the bay leaves.

Purée the soup for a few minutes with an immersion blender, leaving the vegetables slightly chunky for texture.

Adjust the seasonings as needed and serve hot.

Nutrition per Serving

Calories: 383; Fat: 15.0g; Cholesterol: 0mg; Sodium: 283mg; Carbohydrates: 59.0g; Fiber: 7.0g; Sugar: 15.7g; Protein: 10.0g

Bacon Avocado Egg Salad

Makes 4 servings

Ingredients

6 large eggs
5 slices of bacon
1 medium avocado, peeled, seed removed and diced
2 tablespoons plain yogurt
2 teaspoons red wine vinegar
2 teaspoons chives, chopped
Salt, to taste
Pepper, to taste

Directions

In a large pot, add the eggs and enough water to cover them. Bring the water to a boil over high heat and boil for 1 minute. Remove the pot from the heat, cover and let stand for 15 minutes.

Drain and rinse the eggs with cold water then let stand until cool to the touch and then gently remove the egg shells.

In a pan, cook the bacon according to the package instructions until crispy, then crumble the bacon into small pieces and set aside.

Chop the cooled and peeled hard-boiled eggs and place in a bowl.

In a separate small bowl, mix together the avocado, yogurt, red wine vinegar and chives.

Add this mixture to the eggs and gently mix together.

Fold in the bacon and season to taste with salt and pepper.

Cover and refrigerate until ready to serve.

Serve the egg salad on toasted gluten free bread, on top of lettuce, or with chopped vegetables like celery and carrots.

Nutrition per Serving

Calories: 246; Fat: 17.2g; Cholesterol: 290mg; Sodium: 346mg; Carbohydrates: 5.5g; Fiber: 3.4g; Sugar: 1.2g; Protein: 14.6g

Mushroom & Artichoke Pesto Pasta Salad

Makes 6 servings

Ingredients

1 package gluten free spiral pasta
2 tablespoons butter
1 pound button mushrooms, quartered
1 can (14-ounces) quartered artichoke hearts, drained
3 cups fresh basil leaves
3 cups fresh arugula
3 cups fresh parsley leaves
1/4 cup freshly grated Parmesan cheese
2 tablespoons olive oil, divided
Salt, to taste

Directions

Cook the gluten-free pasta according to the package instructions then rinse, let cool, and set aside.

Heat the butter over medium-high heat in a large skillet then add the mushrooms and artichoke hearts and cook, stirring occasionally, until the vegetables are lightly browned, about 6 to 8 minutes.
Remove from heat and let cool.

To make the pesto, combine the basil, arugula, parsley, Parmesan cheese and 1 tablespoon of the olive oil and slowly purée in a food processor. Make sure all the items are chopped but don't purée into a liquid. If the mixture appears too thick, add the remaining 1 tablespoon of olive oil.

Add salt to taste.

Toss together the pasta, vegetables and pesto sauce in a large bowl and chill or serve immediately.

Nutrition per Serving

Calories: 171; Fat: 10.6g; Cholesterol: 14mg; Sodium: 142mg; Carbohydrates: 14.0g; Fiber: 3.7g; Sugar: 2.0g; Protein: 7.1g

Tropical Fruit Salad

Makes 4 servings

Ingredients

1 orange, skin removed and chopped into bite-sized pieces
1 cup diced pineapple
1 cup diced mango
1 banana, peeled and chopped into bite-sized pieces
4 dates, chopped
Shredded coconut (sweetened)

Directions

Combine the orange, pineapple, mango, banana and dates in a large bowl and gently mix together.

Scoop the fruit salad into serving bowls and top with the shredded sweetened coconut.

Nutrition per Serving

Calories: 117; Fat: 0.3g; Cholesterol: 0mg; Sodium: 2mg; Carbohydrates: 30.5g; Fiber: 3.8g; Sugar: 23.1g; Protein: 1.4g

Broccoli Slaw with Red Wine Vinaigrette

Serves 4

Ingredients

1 bag (16-ounces) broccoli slaw
1 cup shredded carrots
1 cup diced tomatoes
1/4 cup olive oil
3 tablespoons brown sugar
3 tablespoons red wine vinegar
1/4 teaspoon salt

Directions

In a large mixing bowl, toss together the broccoli slaw, carrots and tomatoes.

In a separate bowl, whisk together the olive oil, brown sugar, red wine vinegar and salt.

Toss the salad with the dressing then cover and refrigerate until ready to serve.

Nutrition per Serving

Calories: 193; Fat: 13.2g; Cholesterol: 0mg; Sodium: 208mg; Carbohydrates: 18.3g; Fiber: 4.2g; Sugar: 10.8g; Protein: 3.8g

Summer Salad Blend with Blueberry Vinaigrette

Makes 4 to 6 servings

Ingredients

For the Blueberry Vinaigrette

1 cup fresh blueberries
1/4 cup basil, roughly chopped
1/8 cup Balsamic vinegar
1/8 cup olive oil
1/2 teaspoon Dijon mustard
1 teaspoon red onion, minced
1/4 teaspoon garlic, minced
1/4 teaspoon honey
1/4 teaspoon coarse salt (Sea or Kosher)
1/4 to 1/2 teaspoon black pepper

For the Summer Salad Blend

4 cups arugula
1 cup cucumber, diced
1 cup cherry tomatoes, sliced in half
1 cup blueberries
1/2 cup goat cheese, crumbled

Directions

To make the blueberry vinaigrette, purée the blueberries, basil, Balsamic vinegar, olive oil, Dijon mustard, red onion, garlic, honey, salt and black pepper in a blender until smooth.

In a large bowl, toss together the arugula, cucumber, tomatoes, blueberries, and goat cheese.

Drizzle the blueberry vinaigrette over the top of the salad before serving.

Nutrition per Serving

Calories: 160; Fat: 12.0g; Cholesterol: 5mg; Sodium: 150mg; Carbohydrates: 12.0g; Fiber: 2.0g; Sugar: 9.0g; Protein: 3.0g

Side Dishes and Snacks

THE RECIPES

Rosemary Glazed Carrots

Makes 6 servings

Ingredients

2 tablespoons olive oil
1 pound carrots, washed, cleaned and chopped into 1/2-inch pieces
1/2 cup chicken or vegetable stock
2 teaspoons sugar
1 teaspoon chopped rosemary

Directions

Heat the oil over medium heat in a large sauté pan then add the carrots and cook, stirring occasionally, for 5 to 7 minutes.

Add the chicken stock, sugar and rosemary and cook over low heat until the liquid is reduced to a glaze.

Serve immediately.

Nutrition per Serving

Calories: 95; Fat: 5.2g; Cholesterol: 9mg; Sodium: 60mg; Carbohydrates: 8.8g; Fiber: 2.2g; Sugar: 5.0g; Protein: 4.1g

Roasted Asparagus with Chive Dressing

Makes 4 servings

Ingredients

1-1/2 pounds asparagus, trimmed
1 teaspoon olive oil
1/8 teaspoon coarse salt
1/8 teaspoon black pepper
1 tablespoon olive oil
1 teaspoon lemon juice freshly squeezed
1/4 teaspoon lemon zest
1 teaspoon minced chives
1/8 teaspoon black pepper
Salt, to taste
4 ounces goat or blue cheese (optional)
1/4 cup toasted almonds, walnuts or pine nuts (optional)

Directions

Preheat the oven to 400°F and line a baking sheet with foil.

In a large bowl toss the asparagus with the olive oil, salt and black pepper.

Spread out the asparagus on the baking sheet then place in the oven and roast for 10 minutes (up to 15 minutes if you like the spears softer).

While the asparagus is cooking, combine the lemon juice, lemon zest, chives, black pepper, and salt to taste in a small bowl.

Remove the asparagus from the oven then place on a serving plate and drizzle the chive dressing on top.

If using the cheese or nuts, or both, sprinkle over the asparagus prior to serving.

Nutrition per Serving

Calories: 221; Fat: 18.8g; Cholesterol: 21mg; Sodium: 497mg; Carbohydrates: 6.4g; Fiber: 2.8g; Sugar: 2.6g; Protein: 9.8g

Roasted Leeks & Cremini Mushrooms with Balsamic Cream Drizzle

Makes 4 servings

Ingredients

1 pound crimini mushrooms, halved
1 pound leeks, white and light green parts, halved and cut into large sections
1 tablespoon olive oil
1/4 teaspoon salt
1/4 teaspoon black pepper
1/4 cup heavy whipping cream
4 tablespoons balsamic vinegar

Directions

Preheat the oven to 400°F.

In a large bowl, toss the mushrooms and leeks with olive oil, salt and pepper to coat.

Spread out the mushrooms and leeks on a baking sheet then place in the oven and roast for 10 to 15 minutes, or until the leeks soften and the mushrooms brown.

While the vegetables are in the oven, whisk together the heavy whipping cream and the balsamic vinegar and set aside.

Remove the vegetables from the oven and let rest for 2 minutes.

To serve, place the vegetables on a serving dish and then drizzle with the balsamic cream, or serve on the side.

Nutrition per Serving

Calories: 159; Fat: 6.7g; Cholesterol: 10mg; Sodium: 180mg; Carbohydrates: 21.1g; Fiber: 2.8g; Sugar: 6.4g; Protein: 4.7g

Fried Plantains with Mango Chutney

Makes 4 servings

Ingredients

2 tablespoons butter
1/4 cup diced red onion
1 tablespoon chopped fresh ginger
1/2 teaspoon chili powder
1/2 bay leaf
1/4 cinnamon stick
3 ripe mangos, peeled, seed removed and diced
1 tablespoon extra-virgin olive oil
2 teaspoons lime juice
2 tablespoons honey
1/2 teaspoon salt
1/2 teaspoon pepper
Vegetable oil for frying
3 semi-ripe plantains
Salt, to taste

Directions

To make the chutney, heat the butter in a small sauce-pot over medium-low heat then add the red onion, ginger, chili powder, bay leaf and cinnamon stick and cook, stirring frequently, until the onions become translucent and slightly caramel in color, about 10 minutes.

Add the mangos, olive oil, lime juice, honey, salt and pepper and simmer, stirring often, until the mangos are very soft but still hold their shape, about 15 minutes, then remove from the heat and let cool completely.

To make the plantains, fill a large sauce-pot about halfway with vegetable oil and heat over medium-high heat until the oil reaches 350°F.

Peel the plantains and cut them on the diagonal into slices about 1-inch thick then carefully place the plantains in the frying pan and fry until golden on the outside, about 4 to 6 minutes.

Remove the plantains from the hot oil and place on a paper towel to absorb the excess oil.

Place the fried plantains on a cutting board and smash tem to about 1/8-inch in thickness using a flat object such as the bottom of a plate.

Place the flattened plantains back into the hot oil and fry until golden brown on the entire surface, about 3 to 5 minutes.

Remove the plantains from the oil then place them onto a towel and immediately season them with salt.

Place some of the hot fried plantains on the base of a plate and top with the mango chutney.

Nutrition per Serving

Calories: 192; Fat: 9.8g; Cholesterol: 15mg; Sodium: 378mg; Carbohydrates: 28.6g; Fiber: 3.3g; Sugar: 23.4g; Protein: 1.1g

Smoked Paprika Kale Chips

Makes 10 servings

Ingredients

1 bunch lacinato kale, stems removed and torn into large pieces
1 tablespoon olive oil
1/2 teaspoon smoked paprika
1/2 teaspoon salt
1/2 teaspoon pepper

Directions

Preheat the oven to 350°F and line a baking sheet with parchment paper and set aside.

Ensure that the kale is very dry by patting it down with paper towels and let air dry if necessary.

Place the dried torn strips of kale into a large bowl then drizzle the olive oil over the kale and "massage" into the kale until evenly coated.

Add the paprika, salt, and pepper and toss to combine.

Bake for 12 to 15 minutes until dark and crispy.

Let cool.

Nutrition per Serving

Calories: 42; Fat: 1.4g; Cholesterol: 0mg; Sodium: 142mg; Carbohydrates: 6.0g; Fiber: 0.9g; Sugar: 0.0g; Protein: 1.7g

Hot Soft Buttered Gluten-Free Pretzels

Makes 12 pretzels

Ingredients

For the dough

1-1/2 cups warm water
1 tablespoons sugar
2 teaspoons salt
2-1/4 teaspoons quick rise yeast
4 cups gluten free all-purpose flour
4 tablespoons butter, melted
1 gallon water
1/4 cup baking soda

For the topping

1/2 cup hot water
2 tablespoons baking soda
Kosher salt
3 tablespoons unsalted butter, melted

Directions

In the bowl of a standing mixer, combine the warm water, sugar, salt and yeast then let the mixture sit until it becomes foamy, about 5 to 7 minutes.

Add in the gluten free all-purpose flour and melted butter then using the paddle attachment, mix until a smooth dough form.

Rub a large mixing bowl with olive oil and transfer the dough to the bowl. Cover and let the dough rise in a warm place for 30 minutes.

In a large pot, heat the water and baking soda over high heat until it comes to a boil.

Line a baking sheet with parchment paper and spray with non-stick spray.

Roll the pretzel dough into long stick and then fold into a pretzel shape. Or if desired, roll the dough into thick breadsticks, about 4-inches long.

Carefully drop each pretzel or pretzel stick into the boiling water for about 30 seconds. Remove from the water and place on the greased baking sheet. Repeat until all the dough is boiled.

In a small bowl, whisk together the 1/2 cup of hot water and 2 tablespoons of baking soda then brush each pretzel with the mixture and sprinkle the kosher salt on top.

Bake the pretzels for 10 to 15 minutes, or until they are golden.

Remove from the oven and immediately brush with melted butter.

Cinnamon Sugar Soft Pretzels

Combine 1 tablespoon of ground cinnamon and 1 tablespoon of sugar.

After brushing each pretzels with the baking soda and water mixture, sprinkle each with the cinnamon sugar.

Pizza Soft Pretzels

Brush the pretzels with the baking soda mixture, then scatter pepperoni pieces and mozzarella cheese on top and serve with marinara sauce.

Garlic Cheddar Soft Pretzels

Combine 1 tablespoon of garlic powder and 2 teaspoons of salt.

After brushing the pretzels with the baking soda and water mixture, sprinkle each with the garlic salt mixture and top with cheddar cheese.

Nutrition per Serving

Calories: 188; Fat: 5.1g; Cholesterol: 11mg; Sodium: 1,240mg; Carbohydrates: 31.6g; Fiber: 2.1g; Sugar: 1.4g; Protein: 3.3g

Key Lime Shrimp Tacos

Makes 6 servings

Ingredients

3 tablespoons olive oil, divided
1-1/2 pounds raw shrimps, peeled and deveined
1 cup thinly sliced white onion
1 red bell pepper, seeded and thinly sliced
3 cloves garlic, finely minced
1/4 cup chopped cilantro
1/2 cup tequila
1 tablespoon lime juice
1 teaspoon salt
1/2 cup sour cream
18 corn tortillas, heated

Directions

In a large skillet, heat 2 tablespoons of olive oil over medium-high heat then add in the shrimp and cook for 3 minutes, flipping them once during this time. Remove the shrimp from the pan and set aside.

To the same pan, add the remaining 1 tablespoon of olive oil and heat over medium-high heat then add the onions and cook, stirring occasionally, for 5 minutes.

Add in the sliced red bell pepper and cook an additional 3 minutes.

Add in the garlic and cook for 2 more minutes, stirring frequently.

Add in the cilantro and return the partially cooked shrimp to the pan.

Add in the tequila, lime juice and salt, then bring to a simmer and cook for 2 minutes.

Remove the pan from the heat and immediately whisk in the sour cream.

Evenly distribute the shrimp mixture amongst the tortillas and serve with the tri-color salsa if desired (see recipe below).

Nutrition per Serving

Calories: 313; Fat: 11.8g; Cholesterol: 11mg; Sodium: 443mg; Carbohydrates: 36.4g; Fiber: 5.3g; Sugar: 3.1g; Protein: 5.2g

Tri-Color Margarita Salsa

Makes 6 servings

Ingredients

1 cup of finely diced roma tomatoes
1/2 cup finely diced white onion
1/4 cup minced cilantro
1 teaspoon minced jalapeno
1 tablespoon lime juice
1 tablespoon tequila
1/4 teaspoon salt

Directions

Gently mix together the ingredients, then cover and refrigerate until ready to serve.

Smoked Salmon Deviled Eggs

Makes 12 servings

Ingredients

6 large eggs
2 ounces cream cheese, at room temperature
2 tablespoons mayonnaise
1 teaspoon freshly squeezed lemon juice
4 ounces smoked salmon, minced
1 tablespoon capers rinsed, drained, and finely chopped
Salt, to taste
Pepper, to taste
Fresh dill or chives for garnish (optional)

Directions

In a large pot, add the eggs and enough water to cover them. Bring the water to a boil over high heat and boil for 1 minute. Remove the pot from the heat, cover, and let stand for 15 minutes. Drain and rinse the eggs with cold water and let stand until cool to the touch and then gently remove the egg shell.

Gently cut the eggs in half lengthwise then remove the yolks and place them in a small bowl.

Mash the yolks with a fork and then stir in the cream cheese, mayonnaise, lemon juice, smoked salmon and capers.

Add salt and pepper to taste.

Fill the egg whites evenly with the yolk mixture by either piping a rosette into each egg white half with a pastry bag or filling carefully with a spoon.

Garnish with fresh dill or chives, if desired.

Store covered in the refrigerator until ready to serve.

Nutrition per Serving

Calories: 80; Fat: 5.8g; Cholesterol: 100mg; Sodium: 157mg; Carbohydrates: 0.4g; Fiber: 0.0g; Sugar: 0.3g; Protein: 5.2g

Oven Beef Jerky

Makes 10 servings

Ingredients

2 pounds of sirloin, flank steak, or London broil, trimmed of visible fat
2/3 cups low-sodium gluten free tamari soy sauce
1 teaspoon honey
2 teaspoons pepper
1 teaspoon garlic powder
1 teaspoon smoked paprika
1/2 teaspoon ground ginger
1 teaspoon red pepper flakes (optional)

Directions

Trim the visible fat off the beef.

Wrap the beef tightly in plastic wrap and freeze for one hour to help with slicing.

Remove the meat from the freezer and slice along the grain into 1/8-inch thick strips.

Combine the remaining ingredients in a small bowl and whisk to combine.

Place the beef and marinade in a large bag, then seal and gently turn a couple of times to coat.

Refrigerate for 4 to 6 hours, turning after about 3 hours.

Preheat the oven to the lowest setting (150 to 170°F) and place a wire rack on a large, foil line baking sheet and set aside.

Remove the beef from the marinade and place on a paper towel lined plate or board. Cover with additional paper towels and press down firmly to remove as much moisture as possible.

Place the strips on a wire rack ensuring that they do not touch and have a bit or room on each sides for air circulation.

Place the sheet in the oven and use a rolled kitchen towel or wooden spoon to prop open the oven door.

Let the jerky cook for 5 hours and check the doneness. If done, remove and let cool to room temperature. Continue to cook the jerky, if necessary, for an additional 1 to 2 ours.

Nutrition per Serving

Calories: 175; Fat: 5.7g; Cholesterol: 81mg; Sodium: 107mg; Carbohydrates: 1.4g; Fiber: 0.0g; Sugar: 0.8g; Protein: 27.8g

Grain-Free Bread

Makes 10 servings

Ingredients

1/4 cup coconut flour
1/4 cup blanched almond flour
1-1/2 teaspoons baking soda
1/2 teaspoon salt
1 cup unsweetened roasted almond butter
4 eggs, room temperature separated
1-1/2 tablespoons honey
1/4 cup unsweetened almond milk
2-1/2 teaspoons apple cider vinegar

Directions

Preheat the oven to 300°F and line a loaf pan with parchment paper, leaving a bit of overhang on the side. Set aside.

In a large bowl, combine the coconut flour, almond flour, baking soda, and salt then whisk to combine. Set aside.

In a separate bowl, beat together the almond butter, egg yolks, honey, almond milk and apple cider vinegar.

In a stand mixer or using a hand mixer, whip the egg whites until stiff peaks form.

Add the egg yolk and nut butter mixture to the dry ingredients and beat to combine.

Gently fold in the egg whites until fully combined.

Pour the batter into the pan and bake for 45 to 50 minutes or until the bread springs back when touched and a toothpick inserted in the center comes out clean.

Let cool on a wire rack for 10 minutes then remove from the pan and continue cooling.

Nutrition per Serving

Calories: 170; Fat: 13.0g; Cholesterol: 0mg; Sodium: 330mg; Carbohydrates: 9.0g; Fiber: 3.0g; Sugar: 3.0g; Protein: 7.0g

Sandwiches and Burgers

THE RECIPES

Smashed Avocado BLT

Makes 1 sandwich

Ingredients

2 slices gluten free bread, lightly toasted
1/2 avocado, smashed
2 strips bacon, cooked until crispy
1 lettuce leaf
1 slice of tomato
Salt, to taste
Pepper, to taste

Directions

Place the smashed avocado on one side of the bread and top with the bacon, then lettuce and finally the tomato.

Season the sandwich to taste with salt and pepper and top with the other slice of bread.

Nutrition per Serving

Calories: 610; Fat: 38.7g; Cholesterol: 42mg; Sodium: 1,661mg; Carbohydrates: 49.9g; Fiber: 9.0g; Sugar: 1.1g; Protein: 20.2g

Grilled Cheese Sandwich with Caramelized Onions

Makes 1 sandwich

Ingredients

3 tablespoons butter, divided
1 sweet yellow onion, thinly sliced
1 teaspoon sugar
1 slice cheddar cheese
1 slice Swiss cheese
1 slice Monterey jack cheese
2 slices gluten free bread

Directions

Heat 2 tablespoons of butter in a skillet over low heat then add the onions and gently stir to coat.

Sprinkle with sugar and continue to cook on low heat until caramelized, about 1 hour, then let cool.

Heat 1 tablespoon of butter in a non-stick skillet or non-stick griddle over medium-high heat.

Place the cheese slices on one side of the bread and place 1/4 cup of caramelized onions on the remaining side and gently press together.

Cook the sandwich on the hot skillet or griddle until browned and the cheese begins to melt, about 5 minutes per side.

Nutrition per Serving

Calories: 850; Fat: 64.1g; Cholesterol: 172mg; Sodium: 808g; Carbohydrates: 54.3g; Fiber: 13.0g; Sugar: 15.9g; Protein: 28.7g

Apricot Pesto Turkey Melt

Makes 1 sandwich

Ingredients

2 cups fresh basil, loosely packed
1/4 cup chopped macadamia nuts
1/2 cup dried apricots, chopped
1/2 cup olive oil
Salt, to taste
Pepper, to taste
2 teaspoons butter
2 slices gluten free sandwich bread
4 ounces sliced turkey
1 slice smoked gouda cheese

Directions

To make the pesto, place the basil in a food processor and pulse until the leaves are roughly chopped.

Add the macadamia nuts and apricots to the processor and process until a rough paste forms.

With the processor running, stream in the olive oil until the pesto is thick and the oil is incorporated.

Season the mixture to taste with salt and pepper.

Heat a non-stick skillet or griddle over medium high heat.

Butter one side of each slice of bread.

Spread the pesto on to the unbuttered side of the bread slices.

On one slice, place the turkey and the gouda cheese and gently top with the other bread slice.

Place on the hot skillet or griddle and press down with another pan.

Cook for 2 to 3 minutes per side until golden and the cheese is melted.

Nutrition per Serving

Calories: 620; Fat: 41.0g; Cholesterol: 30mg; Sodium: 1,730mg; Carbohydrates: 32.0g; Fiber: 2.0g; Sugar: 8.0g; Protein: 34.0g

Reuben

Makes 1 sandwich

Ingredients

2 slices gluten free bread
3 tablespoons thousand island dressing, divided
2 slices Swiss or gruyere cheese
1/4 cup sauerkraut, drained of excess liquid, divided
4 ounces pastrami or corned beef
1 tablespoon butter

Directions

Spread 1 tablespoon of the thousand island dressing on each slice of bread.

On one slice of bread, add 1 slice of cheese, 1/8 cup of sauerkraut and the pastrami or corned beef.

Add the remaining tablespoon of thousand island dressing on top of the meat and the remaining cheese slice and sauerkraut then top with the other slice of bread and gently press together.

Heat the butter in a non-stick skillet or on a non-stick griddle over medium-high heat.

Once hot, place the sandwich in the skillet or on the griddle and press down with a spatula or light pan until browned on one side, about 2 to 3 minutes. Repeat on the remaining side.

Nutrition per Serving

Calories: 844; Fat: 57.1g; Cholesterol: 182mg; Sodium: 2,102mg; Carbohydrates: 45.2g; Fiber: 11.4g; Sugar: 10.2g; Protein: 48.4g

Roasted Pepper & Serrano Ham

Makes 1 sandwich

Ingredients

2 slices gluten free bread
1/2 large garlic clove, cut in half
1 tablespoons extra-virgin olive oil
1 to 2 ounces thinly sliced Serrano ham
1 ounce shaved Manchego cheese
1/4 cup jarred roasted red peppers, drained

Directions

Toast the bread until crisp and lightly browned.

Rub 1 side of a toast with the garlic clove.

Brush or drizzle the garlic-side of the toasts with the olive oil.

On 1 slice of toast, layer the ham, cheese, and peppers, then top with the remaining slice of toast, garlic-side down.

Cut the sandwich in half and serve.

Nutrition per Serving

Calories: 453; Fat: 30.6g; Cholesterol: 47mg; Sodium: 757mg; Carbohydrates: 37.1g; Fiber: 10.4g; Sugar: 2.0g; Protein: 17.8g

Pulled Pork Tostada with Avocado Sauce

Makes 10 servings

Ingredients

For the Avocado Sauce

1 avocado
4 tablespoons fresh cilantro chopped
2 teaspoons minced garlic
1/2 teaspoon salt
1/4 teaspoon pepper
2 tablespoons olive oil
2 teaspoons white wine vinegar
1/2 teaspoon lime juice
1/4 teaspoon onion powder
1/4 teaspoon garlic powder

For the Tostada

2 packages (16-ounces) of prepared pulled pork
10 crispy corn tortillas
1-1/2 cups shredded mozzarella or Monterey jack cheese
1-1/2 cups diced tomato
2 cups shredded lettuce

Directions

To make the avocado sauce, combine all the ingredients in a food processor or chopper and pulse until a smooth sauce forms.

Heat the pulled pork according to the package instructions and shred using two forks.

For a picnic, pack up all the ingredients in sealed containers.

To assemble the tostadas, spread the avocado sauce over the surface of each corn tostada and top with the pork, cheese, tomatoes and lettuce.

Nutrition per Serving

Calories: 350; Fat: 15.0g; Cholesterol: 45mg; Sodium: 930mg; Carbohydrates: 36.0g; Fiber: 4.0g; Sugar: 15.0g; Protein: 18.0g

Gyro Burgers with Cucumber Yogurt Sauce

Makes 6 servings

Ingredients

For the Cucumber Yogurt Sauce

1 cucumber
2 cups plain Greek yogurt
1/2 cup sour cream
2 tablespoons apple cider vinegar
2 teaspoons salt
1/4 teaspoon black pepper

For the Burgers

1 pound ground lamb
1 cup crumbled feta
1/2 cup finely minced red onion
2 teaspoons salt
1 teaspoon pepper
6 gluten free hamburger buns

Directions

To make the cucumber yogurt sauce, grate the cucumber into a bowl and then drain out all of the liquid.

Place the shredded cucumber pieces into a larger mixing bowl and mix in the Greek yogurt, sour cream, apple cider vinegar, salt and pepper then cover and refrigerate until ready to serve.

Preheat the grill to high heat.

To make the burger, mix together the ground lamb, crumbled feta, red onion, salt and pepper and form the mixture into 6 equally sized patties.

Grill the hamburgers for 4 to 6 minutes on each side or until the internal temperature reaches 165°F.

Serve on gluten free buns with the yogurt sauce.

Nutrition per Serving

Calories: 590; Fat: 31.0g; Cholesterol: 120mg; Sodium: 2,360mg; Carbohydrates: 41.0g; Fiber: 7.0g; Sugar: 11.0g; Protein: 37.0g

Pizza Burger

Makes 6 servings

Ingredients

1 pound lean ground beef
1 cup marinara sauce, divided
2 cups grated mozzarella cheese, divided
1/3 cup finely chopped yellow onion
1/3 cup finely chopped button mushrooms
1 teaspoon garlic powder
1 teaspoon salt
1/2 teaspoon pepper
6 gluten free hamburger buns

Directions

Preheat the grill to high heat.

In a mixing bowl, mix together the ground beef, 1/2 cup marinara sauce, 1 cup grated mozzarella cheese, onion, mushrooms, garlic powder, salt and pepper.

Form the mixture into 6 evenly sized patties and grill for 4 to 5 minutes on each side.

Evenly distribute the remaining marinara sauce and grated mozzarella cheese over each of the burgers and cook for 1 more minute to the desired level of doneness, or an internal temperature of approximately 160°F is reached.

Serve on gluten free hamburger buns.

Nutrition per Serving

Calories: 420; Fat: 18.0g; Cholesterol: 75mg; Sodium: 1,160mg; Carbohydrates: 38.0g; Fiber: 7.0g; Sugar: 7.0g; Protein: 30.0g

Black Bean, Mushroom & Pesto Burgers

Makes 6 servings

Ingredients

1 can (15-ounces) black beans, drained
1 pound Portobello mushrooms
4 cups cooked brown rice, cooled
1/2 cup pesto sauce
1 cup shredded Gruyere cheese
1 egg
1 teaspoon salt
1/2 teaspoon garlic powder
6 gluten free hamburger buns

Directions

Preheat the oven to 375°F and line a baking sheet with parchment paper.

In the bowl of a food processor, combine the drained black beans and mushrooms and pulse 4 to 5 times just until broken up.

Add in the cooled rice, pesto sauce, cheese, egg, salt and garlic powder and pulse until coarse crumbs form.

Form the mixture into 8 equally sized patties, about 1/2 cup each then place onto the prepared baking sheet and bake for 20 to 25 minutes until fully set.

Serve on gluten free buns with the desired garnishes.

Nutrition per Serving

Calories: 670; Fat: 31.0g; Cholesterol: 60mg; Sodium: 1,070mg; Carbohydrates: 82.0g; Fiber: 12.0g; Sugar: 6.0g; Protein: 20.0g

Buffalo Chicken Burgers

Makes 6 servings

Ingredients

For the Buffalo Sauce

2 tablespoons butter
2 tablespoons brown sugar
3/4 cup tomato sauce
5 teaspoons hot sauce
1 teaspoon gluten free Worcestershire sauce
1 teaspoon garlic powder
1/2 teaspoon salt

For the Homemade Bleu Cheese Dressing

3/4 cup milk
1 tablespoon lemon juice
1/2 cup sour cream
1/2 cup mayonnaise
1 shallot, finely minced
1 tablespoon minced garlic
1 teaspoon gluten free Worcestershire sauce
1/2 teaspoon hot sauce
1/2 teaspoon salt
1 cup bleu cheese crumbles

For the Burgers

1 pound ground chicken
3/4 cup bleu cheese crumbles
1/4 cup finely minced red onion
Salt
Pepper
6 gluten free hamburger buns
Carrots, for dressing
Celery, for dressing

Directions

To make the buffalo sauce, in a small saucepot, whisk together the butter and brown sugar over medium heat then continue whisking until the mixture begins to simmer.

Whisk in the tomato sauce, hot sauce, Worcestershire sauce, garlic, powder and salt and cook, stirring constantly, for 3 to 4 minutes. Remove from the heat and set aside. Let cool completely.

To make the bleu cheese dressing, in a mixing bowl, whisk together the milk and lemon juice then let sit for 5 minutes.

To this mixture, add in the sour cream, mayonnaise, shallots, garlic, Worcestershire sauce, hot sauce, salt and bleu cheese crumbles and mix together, cover, and refrigerate until ready to serve.

Preheat the grill over high heat.

To make the burgers, in a large mixing bowl, thoroughly mix together the ground chicken, bleu cheese, red onion and buffalo sauce.

Form the mixture into 6 evenly-sized patties and lightly sprinkle with salt and pepper onto one side of each burger.

Grill the burgers for 5 to 6 minutes on each side or until the internal temperature reaches 165°F.

Serve on gluten free hamburger buns and garnish with the homemade bleu cheese dressing, carrots and celery.

Nutrition per Serving

Calories: 620; Fat: 36.0g; Cholesterol: 130mg; Sodium: 1,970mg; Carbohydrates: 47.0g; Fiber: 7.0g; Sugar: 13.0g; Protein: 29.0g

Entrées

THE RECIPES

Grilled Lemon Chicken

Makes 6 servings

Ingredients

6 boneless chicken breasts
3 tablespoons olive oil
Juice of 2 lemons
1 teaspoon fresh thyme leaves
1 teaspoon dried garlic
1/2 teaspoon salt
1/4 teaspoon pepper

Directions

Place a chicken breast in a plastic bag and pound it with a meat mallet (or in a pinch, a can) until the breast has a uniform thickness. Repeat with all the chicken pieces and set aside in a large bowl.

In a separate bowl, whisk together the olive oil, lemon juice, thyme, garlic, salt and pepper then pour the marinade over the chicken and let it sit in the refrigerator for 4 to 6 hours or even overnight.

Pre-heat the grill to high and then grill up to 7 minutes on each side, depending on the thickness of the chicken breasts, making sure not to overcook.

Serve the chicken as a main course or chop the chicken and serve on top of a salad.

Nutrition per Serving

Calories: 560; Fat: 31.0g; Cholesterol: 85mg; Sodium: 376mg; Carbohydrates: 0.5g; Fiber: 0.1g; Sugar: 0.0g; Protein: 60.6g

Citrus Parsley Confit Crusted Salmon

Makes 4 servings

Ingredients

4 cups water
2 tablespoons sugar
1 teaspoon salt
2 lemons
1/2 cup Italian parsley leaves
1/2 teaspoon salt
2 cups potato chips
1/4 cup butter, cold, cut into 1/2-inch cubes
1 garlic clove, peeled
1-1/2 pounds salmon fillet, cut into 4 equal pieces

Directions

To make the lemon confit, combine the water, sugar and salt in a sauce-pot and bring to a boil.

Make four lengthwise incisions in each of the lemons and add the whole lemons to the pot then lower the heat and simmer for one hour until extremely soft.

Remove from the heat and let cool completely in the pot.

When the lemons are cool, drain then dry them well and slice away the peel. Finely chop the peel and set aside. Discard the fruit.

To make the crust for the salmon, combine the parsley and salt in the bowl of a food processor and pulse until the herbs are finely chopped, then add in the potato chips, butter, garlic and chopped lemon peel and pulse until smooth.

Preheat the oven to 400°F.

Place the salmon on a lightly greased baking sheet.

Divide the crust evenly amongst the 4 salmon pieces and spread across the top of each fillet then bake for 24 to 27 minutes until the fish easily flakes.

Nutrition per Serving

Calories: 680; Fat: 46.9g; Cholesterol: 102mg; Sodium: 1,330mg; Carbohydrates: 37.6g; Fiber: 3.4g; Sugar: 7.3g; Protein: 29.3g

Sweet Italian Sausage & Ricotta Skillet Lasagna

Makes 6 servings

Ingredients

1 package gluten free brown rice spiral pasta
2 tablespoons olive oil
1 cup diced sweet yellow onion
3 cups button mushrooms, thinly sliced
1 pound sweet Italian sausage, casings removed
1 cup diced celery
1 cup chopped carrots
1 tablespoon minced garlic
2 teaspoons dried Italian seasoning
2 cans (14-1/2-ounces, each) tomato sauce
1 tablespoon brown sugar
2 teaspoons salt
1/2 cup part-skim ricotta
2 cups shredded mozzarella cheese, divided

Directions

Cook the gluten free pasta according to package instructions and then drain.

Preheat the oven to 350°F then grease a 9 x 13 glass baking dish and set aside.

Pour the cooked pasta into the baking dish, spread out evenly, and set aside.

Heat the olive oil in a large skillet over medium-high then add the diced yellow onions and mushrooms and cook, stirring occasionally, until the onions are translucent, about 5 to 7 minutes.

Crumble the raw sausage meat and add to the pan and cook, stirring often, until the sausage is cooked through and golden brown.

Add in the celery and carrots and cook for an additional 4 minutes, stirring occasionally.

Add in the minced garlic and cook for 1 additional minute.

Add in the Italian seasoning, tomato sauce, brown sugar and salt then bring the mixture to a boil. Reduce the heat to medium-low and let simmer for 5 to 7 minutes.

Remove the pan from the heat and stir in the ricotta and 1/4 cup of the shredded mozzarella cheese.

Pour the sausage mixture on top of the pasta then spread out into an even layer.

Top with the remaining mozzarella cheese and bake the lasagna for 25 to 30 minutes or until the cheese is bubbly and golden brown.

Nutrition per Serving

Calories: 440; Fat: 21.0g; Cholesterol: 58mg; Sodium: 1,507mg; Carbohydrates: 32.5g; Fiber: 4.8g; Sugar: 9.2g; Protein: 27.2g

Green Curry Tofu & Peas with Brown Rice

Makes 6 servings

Ingredients

1-1/2 cups brown rice
3 tablespoons olive oil, divided
1 medium yellow onion, chopped
1 teaspoon minced garlic
1-1/2 tablespoons green curry paste
1 can (14-ounces) coconut milk
2 tablespoons fish sauce
2 tablespoons brown sugar
1/4 cup chicken stock
1 block (14-ounces) extra firm tofu, cut into 1/2-inch cubes
1 cup frozen green peas

Directions

Cook the brown rice according to the package instruction and set aside.

In a large sauté pan, heat 2 tablespoons of olive oil over medium-high heat then add the onions and cook, stirring occasionally, until the onions are translucent, about 7 minutes.

Add in the garlic and cook 1 additional minute.

Add the remaining 1 tablespoon of olive oil and the green curry paste and swirl the curry paste in the pan until fragrant.

Add in the coconut milk and stir vigorously until the curry paste is thoroughly incorporated. Bring the mixture to a slow boil and then reduce the heat to medium.

Add in the fish sauce, brown sugar and chicken stock then stir until the sugar fully dissolved.

Add in the tofu and green peas then bring the mixture to a simmer and cook for 5 minutes.

Gently stir in the brown rice into the curry mixture before serving.

Nutrition per Serving

Calories: 443; Fat: 27.6g; Cholesterol: 0mg; Sodium: 609mg; Carbohydrates: 38.7g; Fiber: 5.0g; Sugar: 7.5g; Protein: 12.4g

Coffee Rubbed Beef Tenderloin

Makes 4 servings

Ingredients

2 tablespoons Blue Mountain Coffee grounds
1 tablespoon garlic powder
1 teaspoon sea salt
1 teaspoon ground thyme
1 teaspoon chili powder
1/2 teaspoon pepper
2-1/2 pounds beef tenderloin

Directions

To make the rub, combine the coffee grounds, garlic powder, salt, thyme, chili powder and pepper in a food processor or spice grinder and pulse until a fine powder forms.

Rub the spices over the entire surface of the beef tenderloin.

Place the meat in a large bowl then cover with plastic wrap and refrigerate for 2 to 3 hours, or overnight if desired.

Preheat the oven to 425°F.

Heat a large oven-proof skillet over medium-high heat.

When the pan is hot, place the beef in the pan and sear the meat for about 2 minutes on each side.

Once browned, transfer the skillet to the preheated oven and cook for 50 to 60 minutes until the internal temperature reaches 135°F.

Let the meat rest for 15 minutes before slicing.

Nutrition per Serving

Calories: 478; Fat: 20.9g; Cholesterol: 209mg; Sodium: 609mg; Carbohydrates: 2.2g; Fiber: 0.6g; Sugar: 0.6g; Protein: 66.1g

Leek and Portobello Risotto

Makes 4 servings

Ingredients

4 cups chicken or vegetable stock
1/2 cup dry white wine
1 tablespoon unsalted butter
1 cup chopped leeks, white part only
3 cups Portobello mushrooms, chopped
1 cup Arborio rice
1/2 cup grated Parmesan cheese
Salt, to taste
Pepper, to taste

Directions

In a small pot over medium-low heat, combine the chicken stock and white wine then bring to a slow simmer.

In a separate medium-sized pot over medium heat, melt the butter and then add the leeks and mushrooms.

Sauté the leeks and mushrooms until softened, about 5 to 7 minutes, then add salt.

Add the rice to the pot and use a wooden spoon the combine with the fresh vegetables. Cook for 1 minute.

Pour 1 cup of warm stock into the pot with the rice and vegetables then stir to combine and let cook until all the liquid is almost fully reduced.

Continue this process until all the stock mixture has been added to the rice mixture. Keep an eye on the heat level so the rice mixture does not scorch and stick to the bottom of the pot.

Once all the liquid has been absorbed, remove the pot from the burner and stir in the Parmesan cheese.

Add salt and pepper to taste prior to serving.

Nutrition per Serving

Calories: 270; Fat: 8.0g; Cholesterol: 0mg; Sodium: 380mg; Carbohydrates: 35.0g; Fiber: 2.0g; Sugar: 4.0g; Protein: 11.0g

Chicken, Cilantro & Mushroom Enchilada Casserole

Makes 6 servings

Ingredients

3 tablespoons olive oil, divided
1 large sweet onion, diced
1 package (8-ounces) button mushrooms, thinly sliced
4 cloves garlic, minced
4 cups cooked shredded rotisserie chicken
4 cups lightly packed fresh spinach leaves
1/2 cup chicken stock
1 package (8-ounces) cream cheese
1/2 cup chopped cilantro
2 cups grated cheddar Jack cheese blend, divided
1 teaspoon salt
1/2 teaspoon chili powder
18 corn tortillas
1 can (15-1/2-ounces) black beans, drained

Directions

Preheat the oven to 375°F.

Heat 2 tablespoons of olive oil in a large nonstick skillet over medium-high heat then add the onions and mushrooms and sauté, stirring occasionally until the vegetables begin to brown and the onions are soft, about 5 to 7 minutes.

Add the garlic and cook for 1 additional minute.

Add in the remaining 1 tablespoon of olive oil, chicken and spinach and cook, stirring frequently, until the spinach has wilted.

Add in the chicken stock and bring to a boil.

Add the cream cheese and swirl the cheese until it melts completely and a creamy sauce begins to form.

Stir in the cilantro, 1/2 cup grated cheese, salt and chili powder.

Lower the heat to medium-low and let simmer for 3 minutes.

Meanwhile, spray a 9 x 13-inch casserole dish with nonstick spray.

Layer 6 corn tortillas along the bottom of the pan, then pour all of the chicken and spinach mixture on top of the tortillas and spread out in an even layer. Top this layer with 6 more corn tortillas.

Pour the drained black beans over the tortillas to make the next layer, then sprinkle 1/2 cup of grated cheese on top of the beans and then top with 6 more corn tortillas.

Sprinkle the remaining 1 cup of grated cheese on top of the casserole.

Bake for 20 to 22 minutes until the cheese is bubbly and golden brown.

Serve with pineapple guacamole if desired.

Nutrition per Serving

Calories: 722; Fat: 13.0g; Cholesterol: 151mg; Sodium: 1,313mg; Carbohydrates: 92.7g; Fiber: 6.0g; Sugar: 52.6g; Protein: 57.3g

Chicken and Broccoli Alfredo

Makes 6 servings

Ingredients

1 package gluten free corn fettuccini
3 tablespoons butter
1 pound chicken breasts, sliced in thin strips
Salt
Pepper
1 head broccoli, cut into bite sized florets
2 tablespoons olive oil
1 sweet yellow onion, skin removed and cut into thin slices
3 cloves garlic, minced
1/4 cup white wine
2 cups heavy cream
1 cup grated Parmesan cheese
1/4 cup chopped parsley

Directions

Cook the gluten free fettuccini according to the package instructions then drain and set aside.

Heat the butter in a large skillet over medium-high heat.

Season the chicken strips with salt and pepper and then add to the hot butter,

Cook until lightly browned on all sides, about 5 minutes.

Add in the broccoli and cook for an additional 3 minutes.

Remove the chicken and broccoli from the pan and set aside.

In the same pan that was used for the chicken, add the olive oil and heat over medium-high heat then add the onions and cook ,stirring frequently, until the onions are soft and translucent, about 5 to 7 minutes.

Add in the garlic and cook for 1 minute, just until fragrant.

Add in the white wine to deglaze the pan, the once the wine has reduced fully, add in the heavy cream.

Bring to a simmer and reduce the heat to medium.

Whisk in the Parmesan cheese and continue stirring until the cheese has fully melted.

Add back in the chicken and broccoli and bring to a simmer.

Toss in the gluten free fettuccini and parsley and season with additional salt and pepper is desired.

Nutrition per Serving

Calories: 511; Fat: 30.0g; Cholesterol: 132mg; Sodium: 398mg; Carbohydrates: 27.5g; Fiber: 5.2g; Sugar: 4.8g; Protein: 28.1g

Steak & Portobello Mushroom Stroganoff

Makes 6 servings

Ingredients

1 package gluten free corn pasta
3 tablespoons cornstarch
1 teaspoon garlic powder
1/2 teaspoon salt
1/2 teaspoon pepper
1-1/2 pounds round steak, cut into thin strips
3 tablespoons olive oil, divided
2 cups sliced yellow onion
1 pound Portobello mushrooms, sliced
1 teaspoon cornstarch
1-1/4 cups beef stock
1 cup cream of mushroom soup
1 cup sour cream
2 teaspoons Worcestershire sauce
Salt, to taste
Pepper, to taste
Chive, for garnish

Directions

Cook the gluten free pasta according to the package instructions then drain and set aside.

Meanwhile, in a small bowl, mix together the 3 tablespoons of cornstarch, garlic powder, salt and pepper.

Sprinkle this mixture over the strips of steak and toss to coat well.

Heat 2 tablespoons of olive oil in a nonstick pan over medium-high heat then add the coated steak and cook, stirring occasionally, for 5 to 7 minutes until the meat becomes caramelized and browned.

Remove the meat from the pan and set aside.

To the same pan, add the remaining 1 tablespoon of olive oil and heat over medium-high heat then add the sliced onions and Portobello mushrooms and cook, stirring occasionally, for 6 to 8 minutes, or until the onions are translucent and being to brown.

Whisk together the beef stock and 1 teaspoon cornstarch and pour over the vegetables.

Whisk in the cream of mushroom soup and bring the mixture to a boil.

Reduce the heat to medium and whisk in the sour cream and Worcestershire sauce.

Add back in the browned steak and bring the mixture to a simmer.

Season to taste with salt and pepper then serve over the cooked gluten free pasta. Garnish with chives, if desired.

Nutrition per Serving

Calories: 816; Fat: 28.0g; Cholesterol: 249mg; Sodium: 883mg; Carbohydrates: 24.9g; Fiber: 3.4g; Sugar: 7.0g; Protein: 101.6g

Margherita Pizza

Makes 4 individual pizzas

Ingredients

1 recipe no-rise crust (see recipe below)
1 cup pizza sauce, divided
24 small fresh mozzarella balls, divided
2 cups cherry tomatoes, halved and divided
1/2 cup fresh basil, chiffonade
1/4 cup olive oil for drizzling, divided

Directions

Preheat the oven to 450°F and line two baking sheets with parchment paper.

Make the no-rise crust and roll out as directed into 4 rustic shaped pizzas, then spread each pizza with 1/4 cup of pizza sauce, leaving room on the edges for a crust.

Add 6 mozzarella balls and 1/2 cup halved cherry tomatoes to each pizza then drizzle with 1 tablespoon of olive oil.

Bake for 10 to 15 minutes or until golden and the cheese is bubbly.

Top with fresh basil before serving.

Nutrition per Serving

Calories: 790; Fat: 37.0g; Cholesterol: 5mg; Sodium: 1,420mg; Carbohydrates: 97.0g; Fiber: 11.0g; Sugar: 36.0g; Protein: 26.0g

No Rise Pizza Crust

Makes 4 individual crusts

Ingredients

1 cup warm water
1 packet rapid rise yeast
1 tablespoon olive oil
1 tablespoon sugar
2-3/4 cups gluten free all-purpose flour
1/4 cup grated Parmesan cheese
1/2 teaspoon sea salt

Direction

Preheat the oven to 450°F.

In the bowl of a stand mixer, combine the warm water, yeast, oil and sugar and let sit until the yeast is puffy, about 5 minutes.

Meanwhile, whisk together the flour, cheese and salt in a large bowl.

Add half of the flour mixture to the yeast and water mixture and beat on low until well incorporated.

Add the remaining flour mixture and mix until the dough is shaggy but thoroughly mixed.

Turn the dough out onto a floured sheet of parchment and divide into 4 equally sized balls.

Oil your hand and gently roll the balls into discs, then roll out using another floured piece of parchment on top of the dough. Roll into rustic shaped pizzas.

Top as desired and bake for 10 to 15 minutes.

Nutrition per Serving

Calories: 350; Fat: 8.0g; Cholesterol: 5mg; Sodium: 420mg; Carbohydrates: 64.0g; Fiber: 9.0g; Sugar: 6.0g; Protein: 12.0g

Desserts

THE RECIPES

Lemon Blueberry Energy Bites

Makes 16 to 18 servings

Ingredients

1/2 cup almonds
12 medjool dates, pitted
1 teaspoon lemon zest
1 cup dried blueberries
1/2 teaspoon cinnamon
1-1/2 cups shredded coconut

Directions

Place the almonds in a food processor and pulse until broken down into small crumbs.

Add the pitted dates to the food processor and process until a smooth paste forms.

Add the lemon zest, dried blueberries and cinnamon then pulse until combined.

Roll the mixture into small ping-pong sized balls with your hands and then roll the balls in the shredded coconut.

Nutrition per Serving

Calories: 116; Fat: 3.0g; Cholesterol: 0mg; Sodium: 1mg; Carbohydrates: 23.9g; Fiber: 3.8g; Sugar: 16.2g; Protein: 1.5g

Vanilla Rainbow Cake with Cream Cheese Frosting

Makes 12 servings

Ingredients

For the Cakes

1-1/4 cups coconut flour
2 teaspoons baking soda
1 teaspoon sea salt
1 cup butter, softened
1 cup sugar
8 eggs, room temperature
4 egg whites, room temperature
1-1/2 cups milk, room temperature
1 vanilla bean, seeds scraped out or 4 tablespoons vanilla extract
1/2 cup colorful sprinkles

For the Frosting

2 packages cream cheese, softened
1 cup powder sugar
1/4 cup heavy whipping cream
1 teaspoon vanilla extract
Additional sprinkles, for garnish

Directions

Preheat the oven to 350°F and grease two round cake pans then set aside.

Combine the coconut flour, baking soda and sea salt in a large bowl then whisk to combine. Set aside.

In the bowl of a stand mixer, cream together the butter and sugar until fluffy and pale yellow.

Add in the eggs, one at a time, and beat well between each addition.

Add the egg whites and beat to incorporate.

Add the coconut flour mixture in two additions, beating well between each addition.

Add the milk and vanilla bean seeds and beat to incorporate.

Gently fold in the sprinkles to create a swirled appearance and transfer to the baking pans.

Bake for 40 to 50 minutes, or until a toothpick inserted in the center comes out clean and the cake is golden brown.

Let cool then remove the cakes from the pans and let cool completely on a wire rack.

To make the frosting, combine the softened cream cheese and powdered sugar in a stand mixer, then beat well until fluffy and the sugar is fully incorporated.

Add the heavy whipping cream and vanilla-extract and beat for another 1 to 2 minutes, or until fully incorporated.

Place one cake onto a cake stand and place a small amount of the frosting in the middle of the cake then gently spread to the edges with an offset spatula.

Carefully place the other cake on top and frost the top and sides.

Garnish with sprinkles.

Nutrition per Serving

Calories: 480; Fat: 33.0g; Cholesterol: 85mg; Sodium: 760mg; Carbohydrates: 39.0g; Fiber: 4.0g; Sugar: 30.0g; Protein: 9.0g

Strawberry Shortcakes

Makes 12 servings

Ingredients

1/2 cup coconut flour
2 tablespoons blanched almond flour
1/4 teaspoon baking powder
1/2 teaspoon sea salt
4 whole eggs, room temperature
2 egg yolks, room temperature
1/2 cup butter, melted
1/2 cup honey
1 teaspoon vanilla extract
2 egg whites
1 pound strawberries, diced
Whipped cream for garnish

Directions

Preheat the oven to 350°F and lightly grease a muffin tin then set aside.

Combine the coconut flour, almond flour, baking powder and sea salt in a large bowl then whisk to combine and set aside.

In a blender (or using an immersion blender), blend together the 4 eggs plus 2 egg yolks, butter, honey, and vanilla until thin and fully combined, then set aside.

In the bowl of a stand mixer, or using a hand mixer, whip the 2 egg whites until stiff peaks form.

Add the egg yolk mixture to the dry ingredients then whisk well or blend to combine.

Gently fold in the egg whites until fully incorporated.

Divide the batter evenly between the muffin tins and bake for 25 to 35 minutes until golden, or until a toothpicks inserted in the center comes out clean.

Let cool on a cookie rack.

Gently slice the shortcakes in half and fill with a layer of diced strawberries, a dollop of whipped cream and then more strawberries.

Nutrition per Serving

Calories: 160; Fat: 10.0g; Cholesterol: 55mg; Sodium: 180mg; Carbohydrates: 15.0g; Fiber: 2.0g; Sugar: 11.0g; Protein: 3.0g

Cherry Chocolate Truffles

Makes 12 servings

Ingredients

1 cup raw pecans
3/4 cup dried cherries
1 tablespoon coconut oil
1/4 cup vegan cocoa powder
1/4 cup finely shredded coconut

Directions

In a food processor, combine the pecans, dried cherries, and coconut oil and process until well combined.

Roll the mixture in your hands to form 1-inch balls.

Lightly roll the balls in loose cocoa powder and top with the shredded coconut.

Place in the refrigerator for 20 minutes to set.

Serve cold or at room temperature.

Nutrition per Serving

Calories: 94; Fat: 9.2g; Cholesterol: 0mg; Sodium: 2mg; Carbohydrates: 3.5g; Fiber: 3.0g; Sugar: 0.0g; Protein: 1.9g

Lemon Bars

Makes 12 servings

Ingredients

2 cups gluten free all-purpose flour
1/2 cup powdered sugar, plus more for topping
2 sticks butter, each cut into 5 pieces
2 cups sugar
4 eggs, beaten
2/3 cup lemon juice
1 tablespoon lemon zest
1-1/2 tablespoons cornstarch
1 teaspoon baking powder
1/4 teaspoon salt

Directions

Preheat the oven to 300°F.

In the bowl of a food processor, pulse together the gluten free all-purpose flour and powdered sugar, then add in the butter until well blended.

Press the crust into the bottom of a 9 x 13-inch glass baking dish.

Bake the crust for 25 minutes then remove from the oven and set aside.

While the crust is baking, whisk together the sugar, eggs, lemon juice, lemon zest, cornstarch, baking powder and salt.

Pour the filling on top of the crust.

Increase the oven temperature to 350°F and bake the bars for 28 to 30 minutes, or until the filling sets.

Dust with powdered sugar before serving.

Nutrition per Serving

Calories: 311; Fat: 16.8g; Cholesterol: 95mg; Sodium: 183mg; Carbohydrates: 39.6g; Fiber: 0.0g; Sugar: 38.6g; Protein: 2.1g

Double Chocolate Brownies

Makes 100 small servings

Ingredients

Dry Ingredients

3/4 cup all-purpose gluten-free, corn-free flour mix
3/4 cup unsweetened cocoa powder
1 teaspoon corn-free baking powder
1/4 teaspoon baking soda
1/2 teaspoon sea salt
1/2 teaspoon guar gum*
3/4 cup granulated sugar
2/3 cup packed dark brown sugar
1/2 cup chocolate chips

Wet Ingredients

1/2 cup light-tasting corn-free oil of choice
2 large eggs, room temperature
2 tablespoons warm water

** Xanthan gum can be used if tolerated*

Directions

Preheat the oven to 350°F then grease an 8 x 8-inch square or a 9–inch cake pan.

In the bowl of your standing mixer fitted with the paddle attachment, mix all the dry ingredients (except the chocolate chips) until combined.

Add the wet ingredients and mix on medium-low until thoroughly combined.

Stir in the chocolate chips.

Spread the batter into the prepared pan with a wet spatula.

Bake on the center rack for 25 to 30 minutes, or until the top is set and a toothpick comes out a bit gooey.

Let cool in the pan for 1 hour before cutting.

Freeze the leftovers.

Nutrition per Serving

Calories: 325; Fat: 35.9g; Cholesterol: 4mg; Sodium: 16mg; Carbohydrates: 4.3g; Fiber: 0.0g; Sugar: 3.2g; Protein: 0.4g

Chocolate Orange Silk Tart

Serves 6 to 8

Ingredients

Chocolate Shortcake Crust

1/3 cup coconut sugar
2 tablespoons coconut nectar or pure maple syrup
1 teaspoon pure vanilla extract
1/3 cup coconut oil, melted
1 cup flour blend of choice
3 tablespoons brown rice flour
1/4 cup unsweetened cocoa powder
1/2 teaspoon baking powder
1/8 teaspoon fine sea salt
1/2 teaspoon stevia powder

Orange Chocolate Ganache Filling

5 ounces good-quality unsweetened chocolate, chopped
2/3 cup coconut sugar
1 cup full-fat coconut milk
1 teaspoon pure vanilla extract
2 teaspoons finely grated orange zest
20 to 30 drops plain or vanilla-flavor stevia liquid, to taste
Pinch fine sea salt

Directions

Grease an 8-inch tart pan or spring-form pan or line it with parchment paper then set aside.

To make the crust, place the coconut sugar, coconut nectar and vanilla extract in the bowl of a food processor and process until the coconut sugar begins to dissolve, about 30 seconds.

Add the coconut oil and process to blend.

Add the remaining ingredients and process just to combine (the dough should form a ball).

Pat the dough evenly into the bottom and up the sides of the prepared 8-inch tart pan or about 3/4-inch up the sides of the prepared springform pan (if the dough is too soft to stay on the sides of the pan, refrigerate for 5 to 10 minutes and then proceed).

Refrigerate the crust until completely firm, about 30 minutes.

Preheat the oven to 375°F.

Prick the crust several times across the bottom with a fork ten place in the preheated oven and bake for 15 to 20 minutes, or until it just begins to brown on the edges and is puffed and dry in the middle. Allow to cool completely before filling.

To make the filling, place all the ingredients in a medium sized heavy-bottom pot over the lowest possible heat.

Stir constantly until the chocolate melts and the mixture is silky-smooth.

Pour the mixture over the cooled crust and let cool to room temperature.

Chill for at least 6 hours or overnight before serving.

Nutrition per Serving

Calories: 390; Fat: 19.5g; Cholesterol: 0mg; Sodium: 88mg; Carbohydrates: 53.9g; Fiber: 2.4g; Sugar: 32.9g; Protein: 3.6g

Banana Cupcakes with Banana Buttercream and Chocolate Glaze

Makes 8 cupcakes

Ingredients

1 cup banana purée (about 2 medium bananas)
2/3 cup coconut sugar
10 drops plan stevia extract (optional)
2 tablespoons flax meal
2 teaspoons pure vanilla extract
1/2 cup milk of choice
2 teaspoons freshly squeezed lemon juice
3 tablespoons sunflower oil or light-tasting oil of choice
1-1/4 cup flour blend of choice
1/3 cup sweet rice flour
1 teaspoon baking powder
1 teaspoon baking soda
3/4 teaspoon xanthan gum
1/8 teaspoon salt

Directions

Preheat the oven to 350°F and grease 8 muffin cups or line them with paper liners.

In a small bowl, mix the banana, sugar, stevia, flax meal, vanilla, milk and lemon juice then whisk in the sunflower oil.

In a large bowl, sift together the flour blend, sweet rice, baking powder, baking soda, xanthan gum and salt.

Add the wet mixture to the dry mixture and stir just to combine.

Using a large ice cream scoop or 1/3 measuring cup, fill the prepared muffin cups two-third full.

Place the cupcakes in the preheated oven and bake for 25 to 35 minutes, or until a toothpick inserted in the center of the cupcake comes out clean. Rotate the pan halfway through the baking.

Allow the cupcakes to cool in the pan for 5 minutes then remove to a rack and let cool completely.

Frost with the Banana Buttercream Frosting and decorate with the Chocolate Glaze, if desired (see recipes below).

Banana Buttercream Frosting

Ingredients

1 cup raw coconut butter (not coconut oil), gently melted
1 ripe banana
1/4 cup coconut nectar or 3 tablespoons agave nectar
1 teaspoon pure vanilla extract
20 to 30 drops plain or vanilla stevia extract, to taste
1/8 to 1/4 teaspoon ground turmeric, (optional for color)
Rice milk or milk of choice, as needed

Directions

Place all the ingredients in the bowl of a food processor and process until smooth and creamy.

If necessary, add the rice milk, about 1 tablespoon at a time, to achieve the desired spreading consistency.

Chocolate Glaze

Ingredients

2 ounces good-quality unsweetened chocolate, chopped
1 teaspoon coconut oil or flavorless vegetable oil of choice
20 to 40 drops plain or vanilla liquid stevia, to taste

Directions

Place the chocolate and oil in a small heavy-bottom pot and melt over the lowest heat possible, stirring constantly.

Add the stevia to taste, stirring to blend.

Drizzle over the cupcakes.

Nutrition per Serving

Calories: 226; Fat: 13g; Cholesterol: 1mg; Sodium: 118mg; Carbohydrates: 28g; Fiber: 4g; Sugar: 28.4g; Protein: 3g

Chocolate-Grasshopper Parfaits

Serves 6

Ingredients

Chocolate Mousse

1 (12-ounce) can full-fat coconut milk
1 large ripe avocado, peeled and cut in chunks
1/4 cup unsweetened cocoa powder
6 tablespoons coconut sugar
Pinch fine sea salt
1 teaspoon pure vanilla extract
40 to 50 drops plain or vanilla-flavor stevia liquid, to taste
1 teaspoon xanthan gum

Mint Mousse

1 (12-ounce) can full-fat coconut milk
1 large ripe avocado, peeled and cut in chunks
30 to 40 fresh mint leaves, to taste
Pinch fine sea salt
3/4 teaspoon pure peppermint extract
20 to 30 drops plain or vanilla-flavor liquid stevia, to taste
1 teaspoon pure vanilla extract
1/2 teaspoon xanthan gum

Directions

To make the Chocolate Mousse, place the coconut milk, avocado, cocoa powder, coconut sugar, salt, vanilla extract and stevia in the bowl of a blender and process until the mixture is perfectly smooth and silky.

Sprinkle the xanthan gum over the mixture and blend to incorporate.

Remove to a bowl and refrigerate while you prepare the Mint Mousse.

Wash and dry the blender.

To make the Mint Mousse, place the coconut milk, avocado, mint leaves, salt, peppermint extract, stevia and vanilla extract in the bowl of a blender and process until the mixture is perfectly smooth and silky.

Sprinkle the xanthan gum over the mixture and blend to incorporate.

Use immediately to assemble the parfaits.

Beginning with the mint mousse, alternate the layers of mint and chocolate mousse, ending with a layer of chocolate. Be sure to cover the mint mousse completely to seal out any air.

Garnish with cacao nibs or shaved bittersweet chocolate and dairy-free whipped topping, if desired.

Nutrition per Serving

Calories: 298; Fat: 24.0g; Cholesterol: 0mg; Sodium: 61mg; Carbohydrates: 20.0g; Fiber: 6.0g; Sugar: 16.5g; Protein: 3.0g

Chocolate Avocado Muffins

Serves 10 to 12

Ingredients

2 cups gluten free multi-grain flour blend or all-purpose flour blend of choice
1/2 cup unsweetened cocoa powder
1/2 cup sugar
3 teaspoons baking powder
1/2 teaspoons xanthan gum (omit if already in your flour blend)
1/2 teaspoon ground cinnamon
1/4 teaspoon salt
1 cup chocolate hemp milk or chocolate milk of choice
6 tablespoons coconut oil, softened, or oil of choice
1 teaspoon pure vanilla extract
1/2 cup avocado purée (about 1 medium avocado)
1/2 cup chocolate chips (optional)

Directions

Preheat the oven to 350°F and lightly grease a muffin pan.

Combine the flour blend, cocoa powder, sugar, baking powder, xanthan gum, cinnamon and salt in a bowl. Break up any lumps of cocoa powder then set aside.

Combine the milk, coconut oil and vanilla extract in a large mixing bowl.

Blend on medium speed for about 2 minutes. The coconut oil will be a little bit lumpy.

Scrap down the bowl as needed.

Add the avocado purée and blend another 2 minutes.

Add the dry ingredients and blend until smooth.

Stir in the chocolate chips, if desired, by hand.

Pour the batter evenly into the prepared muffin cups then place in the preheated oven and bake for 22 to 24 minutes, or until a toothpick inserted comes out clean.

Nutrition per Serving

Calories: 214; Fat: 10.0g; Cholesterol: 0mg; Sodium: 151mg; Carbohydrates: 31.0g; Fiber: 3.0g; Sugar: 15.3g; Protein: 2.0g

Conclusion

Switching to a gluten free diet is a big lifestyle change and does take time to get used to. Many people feel deprived when first going on a gluten free diet. However, it is important to stay positive and focus on all the great foods you can eat. I hope that the recipes I have shared have pleasantly surprised you and demonstrated the wide variety of gluten free meals that are available. Many of the ingredients in these recipes can be found at specialty grocery stores that sell gluten free foods. If you can't find them in your area, check with a celiac support group or go online.

If you are new to a gluten free diet, it's a good idea to consult a dietitian who can answer your questions and offer advice about how to avoid gluten products while still maintaining a healthy and balanced diet.

If you enjoyed this cookbook, then you may also enjoy my other, non-gluten-free recipe books:

- Vegetarian Slow Cooker Recipe Book: 30 Easy Set It & Forget It Meals
- Pressure Cooker Recipe Book: Fast Cooking Under Extreme Pressure
- Slow Cooker International Cooking: A Culinary Journey of Set It & Forget It Meals
- 5 Ingredients 15 Minutes Prep Time Slow Cooker Cookbook: Quick & Easy Set It & Forget It Recipes
- Vegetarian Slow Cooker Recipes: Top 71 Quick & Easy Vegetarian Crockpot Recipe Book
- Vegetarian Pressure Cooker Recipe Book: 50 High Pressure Recipes for Busy People

- 4 Ingredients or Less Cookbook: Fast, Practical & Healthy Meal Options

- Satisfying Slow Cooker Meals and More

For more information about myself and to enjoy more amazing recipes, please visit the following sites:

- Maria Holmes author page at www.Amazon.com

- www.holmescookedmeals.com website

- Holmes Cooked Meals Facebook page

I will be writing and publishing more cookbooks in the future, so please stay tuned. But for now, I would like to thank you for helping me and supporting my efforts to share my passion for cooking.

Thank you!

Index

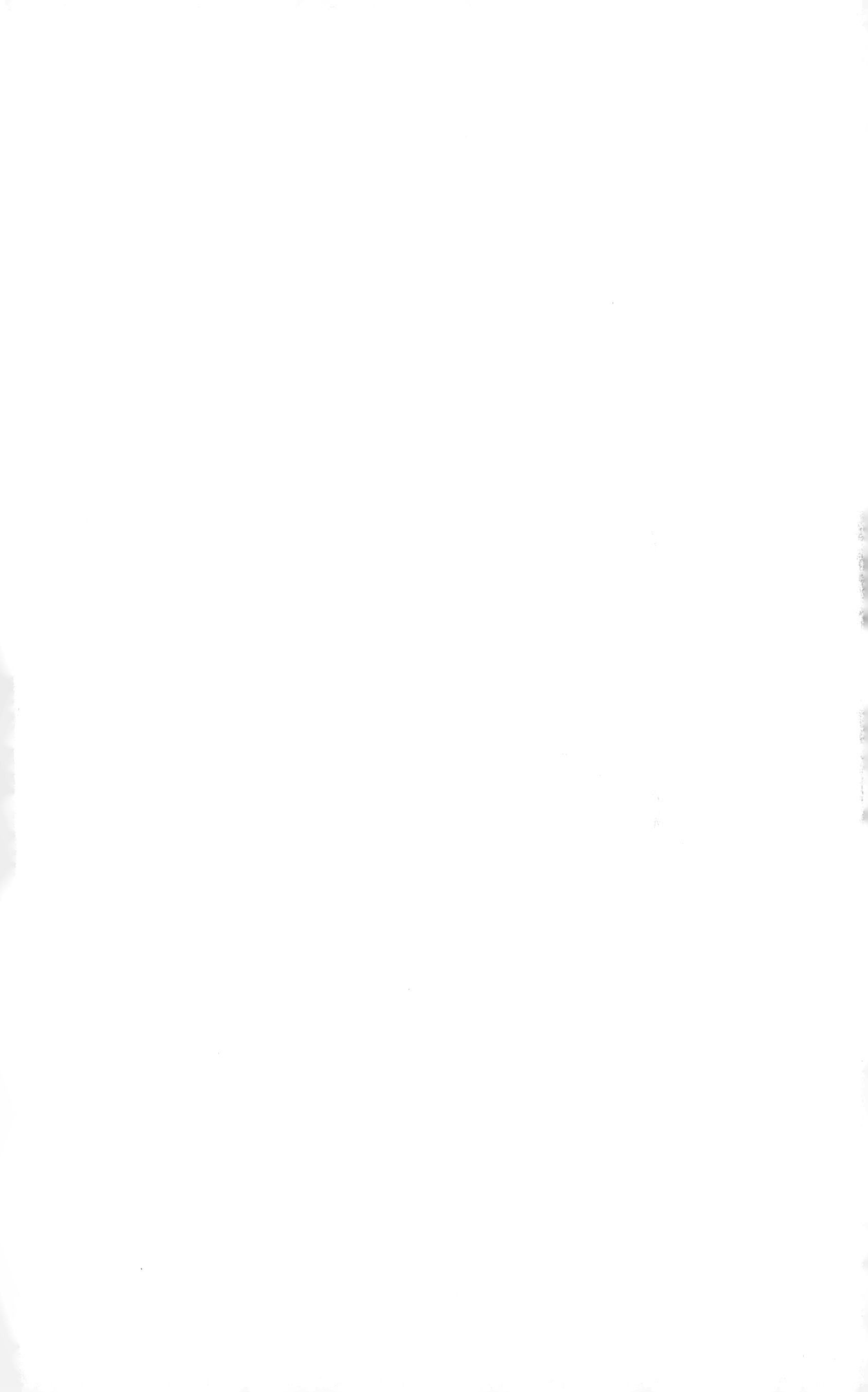

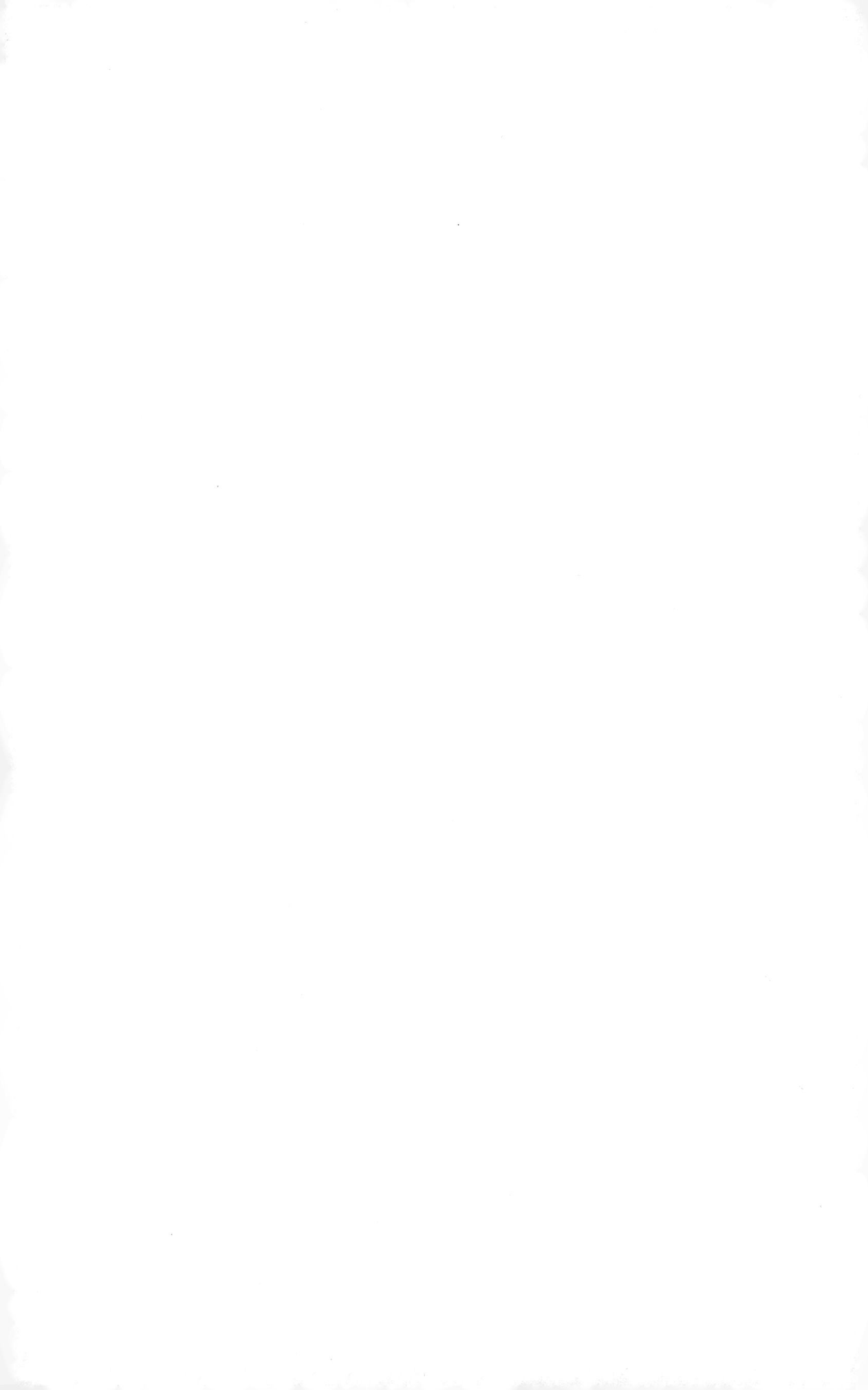

Printed in Great Britain
by Amazon.co.uk, Ltd.,
Marston Gate.